It Will Not Last the Night

I0563740

Sid Prise

chipmunkapublishing
the mental health publisher

Published by
Chipmunkapublishing
PO Box 6872
Brentwood
Essex CM13 1ZT
United Kingdom

http://www.chipmunkapublishing.com

Chipmunkapublishing gratefully acknowledge the support of Arts Council England.

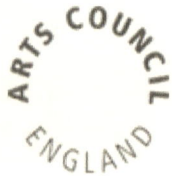

Author Biography

Sid Prise is a writer and activist born in 1972 in Chicago. Sid was diagnosed with Undifferentiated Schizophrenia in 1997, following a prolonged mental and emotional crisis culminating in hearing voices, which he deals with to this day. He has been writing seriously since 1994, and published his first novel, True Faith, in 2003. More of his writings are published online at www.smallaxebooks.com. He resides with his partner, Kathy, and their friends in a collective house in Chicago.

Sid Prise

This novel, *It Will Not Last the Night,* takes place in the years between the Great War and the rise of the Nazis in Germany, the era famous and infamous as "The Weimar Republic." It portrays a small group of radical people and their fight against the tyrannies of fascism, communism, and the capitalist status quo in the period. It is meant as a celebration of one of the greatest eras of human freedom in modern history, which thrived in the midst of a decade of unprecedented political and cultural turmoil. It is meant also as an alternative myth to the well-known narrative that the decadence of the 1920s somehow "led" to Nazism, as the well-deserved unpleasant hangover to the drunken merriment of the decade. That narrative is no less a myth for its widespread acceptance than the myth of the following pages, which celebrates the positive achievements and the unrealized potentials of the Weimar era, rather than regretting its glory. The "decadence" of the 1920s forged bold new ways of living, experiments in social, artistic, and sexual liberation that have yet to be surpassed by the radicalisms of our time. This novel offers a glimpse at the glory of the era, a history that was buried by its fascist successors, and continues to be all but unknown to us today. It has been my exciting task not only to research what escaped the Nazis' bonfires, but to imagine the kinds of characters who might have flourished in such a thrilling time, in whose narratives much of the lost history lives again. The "perversions" the protagonists delight in, defying the Victorian pruderies of the century before, are not inconsequential to the overall project of liberation they profess in every other aspect of their lives. Then, as now, sexual freedom, in all its dark and delicious variations, is a cornerstone of human freedom. And then, as now, sexual variation from hetero-normative strictures imposed by authoritarian societies may threaten those who fear their own sexuality, or in some way defend the mores imposed by authority. It may well threaten those who look with guilt to this era, and to the freedom it realized. This novel is not meant for the fearful, nor the guilt-ridden. It is meant for those who long to know their own freedom and queerness and radicalism is not the province of just the last forty years of the "modern" or "postmodern" world, but has antecedence in the lives of those who are no longer with us—yet still inspire many of us today. It is my hope that the novel will inspire many more.

A note on my use of German phrases and word-forms: Many people identified themselves as being of a "third" gender in the Weimar era—many more than most contemporary folk might appreciate. Whilst I've not found a specific pronoun predominantly used by "intermediate" or "inverted" gendered people in the literature of the time, it is possible to imagine that these folk had their own language to refer to themselves and to others they'd identify in kindred ways, just as contemporary gender-nonconforming folk do today. Most of their literature, as most of the people that read and made it, did not survive the bonfires and crematoria of the Nazi era; so we shall probably never know for sure what words they used, or even if they used the same ones from different queer community to community, queer individual to individual. But the contemporary words ze and hir that people outside the gender binary today sometimes use in the English language to identify themselves descend, according to many queer theorists, from the words sie and ihr, German pronouns which can be translated into the English as either "she/her," "it," or "they," depending on their contexts. In the interest of historical and cultural specificity, I have used these German words in the instances where characters identify so strongly with a third, "intermediate" or "inverted" gender, that they disdain more conventional gender categories. The German word selbst, which means "oneself" when used as a pronoun, is also used, in cases when the character needs to be referred to in a reflexive way. At the suggestion of my friend, Alexander Bokholdt, a fluent German-speaker as well as English-speaker, I have tried to render the object-words along with these pronouns as full German phrases, translating them into their English equivalents in the manner of a bilingual person who would offer the reader or hearer the choice of which language to use. When possible, I've used German words that might function as cognates, hinting at the English words that would complete the sentences. And there are instances, too, where I left German words untranslated, but give enough context, I hope, to allow the words or phrases to be understood. I would also note that many of the characters in this novel are themselves multi-lingual, and at any moment might be *thinking* in German, or English, or French, or Spanish, or in several other languages and dialects. I have done my best to let the reader know in what language(s) the characters are speaking at any given time. My apologies in advance for any confusion.

Many people helped me write this book, many resources. Particularly, I'd like to thank my teacher, Dr. William A. Pelz, a fine specialist in the history of German Socialism, for situating me in a historical context where I could learn and process the details of this time period into a coherent narrative. I'd like to thank also the contemporary writer Mel Gordon for his wonderful recent popular books about the Weimar era, as well as the scholarly authors Karl Eric Toepfer and Maud Lavin for their works about the arts of the era, and Pierre Broue for his excellent work on the political trends of the time. I would also thank the writers and composers of the classic texts of the time itself, notably Christopher Isherwood, Jean Genet, Berthold Brecht, Kurt Weill, Hannah Höch, John Heartfield, George Grosz, Josie Miles, Raoul Hausmann, Harry Reser, Louis Armstrong, Alban Berg, Georg Büchner, Anna Elisabet Weirauch, Radclyffe Hall, and Lucie Delarue-Mardrus. I wish additionally to acknowledge my debt to the political luminaries of this era, notably Karl Liebknecht, Rosa Luxemburg, Marcus Garvey, W.E.B. Du Bois, Paul Eluard, Andre Breton, Louis Aragon, Emma Goldman, Erich Mühsam, Rudolf Rocker, Bruno Rizzi, Milovan Djilis, Nestor Makhno, and Voline. I'd thank as well such contemporary artists as Chumbawamba, World Inferno Friendship Society, The Cabaret of the Nameless and its founder, Madame Betty Devoe, and the film maker Liz Rosenfeld for keeping the spirit of the Weimar '20s and '30s alive. But most of all, I'd like to thank my friends Alexander Bokholdt, Kathryn Rosenfeld, Tyler, and Rugrat for helping me edit this book, for advising me, and for giving me insight into historical and contemporary German culture which I otherwise might have missed. And finally, thank you to all the wonderful people, living and dead, who inspired the characters herein.

Chapter 1

It was a crisp autumn morning in the year 1922, a strange day which featured every season in its passing. The earliest morning, before the dawn, had seen a frost come over the Berlin streets and alleyways, an icy dew that hinted of the coming winter. But by the time the demonstration formed fully on the streets outside the Reichstag, and the chanting took the throats of the leaders of the various factions of the Left in the young and already endangered republic's city, a wave of warm air, unseasonable and almost jarring in its sudden sultriness, wafted over the crowd of thousands from the east, making everyone feel they'd dressed too heavily. People squirmed sweatily in their greatcoats, or, in the case they had no greatcoat (which was many, many), they found even their threadbare jackets, sweaters, dresses and skirts uncomfortable. Had this been another era, or another place, the mob of demonstrators might have proceeded into brazen nakedness on the straße, right there before God and country, and turned their angry urge to storm the Reichstag into a carnal panic of Dionysian proportions. But, as it was, most people were content to be discontented, their leaders shouting their slogans, their ranks cheering and roaring approval or disapproval for what was said, and the hope among them all was that somehow, all this marching and roaring might amount to something more in line with their general feeling of rage.

Hope, and rage. One fed off the other. This time, this place. It was fairly bursting with both, just a few years after the Great War had finally ended, after claiming the lives of millions, and the regency of more than one government. To the east, Russia was fighting to save its revolution, and in the streets of this city, men were battling either for its honour, or against it. Skulls were being cracked, bones broken, blood spilt. And yet, there was hope in it all. Somehow, some new phoenix was struggling to emerge from the ash; just no one knew what name that phoenix would take, what hue its feathers would have, what banner it would carry in its sharp and certain talons. And not everyone could even agree that the ash would not just stay ash, that German, European, even World Civilisation itself, would not just sink into ruin—now, and forever.

But most hoped for that phoenix. Most concluded that ruin was not the fate of humanity. After all, the war had ended, and life had gone on. What was incumbent upon them all was to figure out exactly how to rebuild, in what shape, which direction, and that uncertainty was as damning and exhilarating as anything they'd ever felt in their lives.

Theodor Priser was one who hoped that phoenix had already arisen, in that land to the east, the direction of the warming wind. Strong and lean in his grey overalls and black leather cap, affixed with the red star he'd worn since he was barely more than a boy, he was of the tendency they'd named after Spartacus. A group still forming, still struggling to extricate itself from the great Social Democracy that had been workers' advocates since back in the nineteenth century, but had betrayed those workers (said many; said Theodor) by supporting the recent monstrous war, in which the workers of Germany and Austria were pitted against their comrades in France and England, leaving fields of mud and death where once flowers bloomed, all over Europe. No revolutionary worker could stand with the SPD any more, Theodor concluded, and though he was young, nineteen years, just turned last spring, he'd pledged his life to the newly forming KPD, the Communists, and stood with the new Third International, instead of the bankrupt, "yellow" Second. But unlike his comrades, he saw no great need to shun the Social Democrats, those who for their own reasons still held up the three spears of its banner instead of his own hammer and sickle, and he'd been among those who had organized this demonstration, a united front with them, the Independent Socialists, the Communist Workers' Party, and some of the anarchist groups, to stand against the government and the fascists. For the fascists, he thought, were greater threats to Germany, to German workers, and all working people round the world, than any misguided brethren could ever be.

In this, young Theodor was not in the majority, on either side of the divide. SPD and KPD were fighting in the streets, and the ultra-lefts and the anarchists, ever disruptive, were fighting them both. Meanwhile, the remnants of the disbanded Frei Korps and the new National Socialists (who were "socialist" only in their ironic name) were literally killing people, of all these persuasions, and the Weimar government was doing very little to stop them. Indeed, this was one of the points of unity among the different sects of the Left, and the purported reason for today's gathering. Just days after the government of Italy named the Fascist Mussolini its prime minister, the first government in Europe to fall to the Absolute Right, the threat of the Rightists here was all the more ominous. A united front against fascism could end all this sectarian squabbling, and the better world they'd all fought for in their separate ways could finally come to be. Theodor had high hopes for the demonstration, and the march to follow, which was sufficiently strong to dissuade the Bullen and the Nazis from doing anything to harm them.

Or, so he thought . . .

The workers and their sympathizers marched down the straβen by the thousands away from the Reichstag, into the working class neighbourhoods of the east, their voices raised in rousing choruses of "The Internationale," the anthem that had come out of the Paris Commune of more than two generations before—when all workers who were moved to revolt marched together under the same red flag, regardless of the particular politics that had evolved to divide their descendants—when all rebels sang, in the same triumphant voice—*A BETTER WORLD'S IN BIRTH!* Just at the moment when the chorus thundered that verse a second time, echoing throughout the slums of the Alexanderplatz, overwhelming the bustle and the traffic and rising with the sultry gales from the east—a great company of hundreds of armed, mounted police began charging into them from all sides. People scattered, shouting, calling on each other to resist. But there was no resistance. People who remained in the centre of the street were buffeted and trampled by the horsemen, and it was all people could do to maintain themselves, let alone keep those red flags waving. Theodor was separated from his comrades in the Youth Brigade, and found himself running for his life into an alleyway.

That's when he saw her.

She'd run there, too. A few of her comrades were near her, but they took flight, leaving her to fend for herself, there in a darkened door frame.

"Come on!" she called to Theodor from the door frame, seeing some cops coming out of the main street into the alley. "Come on—over *here!*"

Theodor did not have time to reason this out. A comrade was a comrade, even if they weren't KPD, which this fraulein evidently wasn't. He hurried across the alley, and stood beside her.

"Quick!" she ordered—"Kiss me!"

"What?" Theodor asked, but she did not wait for his reluctance to frustrate her plan. She curled up next to him, putting up a leg up on the door frame, round his waist, and pressed in, as if she were a grasshopper prostitute, getting him off in the alley because there was nowhere else to be.

Theodor began to understand, and kissed her deeply. Only then did he really reflect on what she looked like.

She was dressed very modern, with a short, tassel-fringed black skirt going down no further than her knees, long, poisonous green leather boots laced up tight halfway up her calves, with white ribbons making stylized bows on top. Her body was thickly attractive, curvy and supple, hot against his. Her face was bright olive and rounded, her kohl-streaked eyes somewhere between blue and grey, and her hair, cut short in a *Bubikopf* pageboy-style, tapered on the sides, a little longer in front, peeked from beneath a stylish black cloche, a colour so red that it actually bordered on the pink. Her arms were rounded at the shoulders, dressed in a white, false-ermine fur, but otherwise bare, with a skimpy, lacy, almost diaphanous black blouse, her breasts beneath its folds the gentle curves of a modest Venus De Milo. They pressed sharply against Theodor's lean chest as she kissed him, as if she were enjoying the little deception. Some polizei galloped by, but they didn't give the couple a second glance. A prostitute and her john, they concluded, or some young lovers' tryst. They didn't have time for such things.

The woman opened her eyes, glanced sideways as she kissed Theodor, then closed them again. After a moment, the two fell away, though they still stood quite close in the door frame.

"We'd best stay here a minute or two," she said, looking away, down the alley toward the straβe. "More pigs might come."

"Right," said Theodor. "What's your name?"

She looked at him and chuckled a little.

"You like to know the names of gals ya kiss, huh?"

Theodor smiled.

"Usually, yeah."

"Well, my name's Katharina. What's yours?"

"Theodor."

"Huh. Sexy name."

"Thank you. I've always liked your name, too."

"Well, then—"

—And she kissed him quickly again, her leg up suggestively, as more Bullen rode by. As before, they went on without notice. The noise from the street was dying down. People were being recovered, or arrested, or what-have-you, and the march was effectively over. Still, it made sense to stick to their subterfuge for a few more moments at least, and they did just that. Kissing was a wonderful decoy; Theodor wondered why he'd never thought of it before.

She giggled at length, when the dangers had passed, and said, "You're probably not safe on the streets, now. Neither am I, alone. . . . Say, liebling, ya wanna come up to my place? Just till the heat dies off?"

Theodor chuckled. This was the strangest way yet he'd been introduced to a girl, and he said so. She just shrugged off the comment, as if there was nothing really all that strange about it. He assented to her offer, and the two began to walk down the alleyway.

"I was a little afraid I'd hafta fuck you, Theodor," she said coyly over her shoulder, "just to make it look good. Tell me, suβe, would you have minded that?"

Theodor answered this with a chuckle, at first light and nervous, then, as he thought about it, a hearty one. Well, then! They walked through alleys nearly the whole way, in a jerky, roundabout path toward a seedier neighbourhood of the city, on the outskirts of the Alex, talking a little, but mostly suspending discussion till they could get somewhere safe.

They did learn a little about each other, though. Katharina was an anarchist, attached to some group or other that Theodor had not heard of (though admittedly, in his circles, one did not really bother knowing much about anarchists). She was less attached to "groups" than he was. He imparted that he was a Spartakist, a Communist, and Katharina didn't seem at all surprised. It was evident, she said, in the conservative cut of his sandy-blonde hair, in the drabness of his overalls (she used nicer words to say this, but this is what she said). Theodor was not offended; indeed, he himself had often wondered at the conservatism of his class, or, rather, the conservativeness of those who would shape it. There was something in Communism that seemed to disdain the individuality of attire, that scorned fashion, and though he did not really *like* this, he found himself unconsciously falling in step with it. Besides, if Katharina really meant harm, she could have said far worse.

Still, Theodor understood that conservatism on a level, too. It had to do with sobriety, seriousness. Anarchists (from what little he knew of them) seemed much less sober, far less serious. They either seemed the kind to throw bombs indiscriminately into cafés full of innocent strangers, or the kind that would confuse and bore them with offbeat art exhibitions and queer puppet shows. Like those clowns over there, he smiled to himself, haranguing some

13

drunks on the corner with nonsensical leaflets as Theodor and Katharina approached them, clowns on stilts. They were laughing, and taunting, and cheering the crowd of drunks as if *they* were *their* entertainment, as if the half dozen clowns were an audience of curious onlookers for the show the dreary drunks were putting on for *them*. A few even tossed a few coins at the drunks amidst their weird leaflet cartoons, as well as to the soberer workingmen who were pushing past, gruffly trying to get home after their long day's labours.

"Bravo!" one of them cheered—"Very, very clever! How you stumble like that!"

"And how you trudge like that!" laughed another, tossing a pfennig at a man who had shoved past him grumpily. "Very artful! How studied, your miserableness! You should give me some lessons in that, mein herr!"

Katharina laughed, and exchanged greetings with one of the fellows, a fellow no older than Theodor, skinny, sharply-faced, who smiled through wire-rimmed spectacles. He winked at her, and blew her a kiss as they passed.

"That's Erik Boom!," she chuckled to Theodor parenthetically—"I think I'm in *love* with that boy, liebling."

"That fellow?"

"Why? Not your type?"

"Well . . . no—no. I would say not."

"A little skinny, I know. But you should see 'is act. He's a *contortionist*, darling—what that boy can do with his arms and legs!—and all on a rope, suspended from a bridge, thirty feet over the river—"

"—Yes?"

"*Well*, darling. Any boy worth his salt should know how to move well whilst in suspension . . ."

Theodor didn't really know what that meant, but he laughed it off. He looked back to the stilt-walkers, shaking his head a little at them. *That's* what he thought of anarchists, he chuckled in a kind of wisdom, crumpling and tossing away the leaflet he'd taken from one of them obliviously, a parody Agitprop exhorting workers to steal bananas for the Revolution. He saw the fellow Erik stilt-walk into the straße, smile to his comrades, and spill something onto the pavement from a little handbag. Then they all ambled quickly off. A squad car flew by a few seconds later, and Katharina and Theodor ducked into another alley. The loud boom of a tire blow-out shot out like a pistol, and Katharina laughed as the car careened off the straße onto the pavement, the Bullen getting out and cursing the pile of nails and broken glass and oily banana peels that had been left somehow in the middle of the thoroughfare. Theodor could not help but join her giggling.

Theodor and Katharina finally got to her flat, which was located on a little side street, in an area of town that was run-down in an industrial and, to Katharina, picturesque way. A factory, old, disused, a relic of the munitions industry during the War, sat directly across from her tenement, and otherwise the street sat sadly derelict but for a little tavern with one small, oddly-curtained window, tinted a garish red in a greenish, inner gloom. This, Katharina informed him, was a lesbian bar, which Theodor, though a lifelong Berliner, had never known before. He knew the district well enough, having been raised on a similar street, similarly sad, just a few miles south. But a bar just for lesbians seemed to him an oddity, though a not unwelcome one.

"Have you been in there much?" he asked.

Katharina smiled a wisely impish smile, turning her head as they walked up some rickety steps through a darkened stairwell, with the sounds of a screaming mother wrangling with children in Polish, a jazz combo cuing up for practice, and an old man laughing hysterically, apparently all alone, during their three floor assent, and said, "Of course, darling! Many, *many* times . . ."

Theodor did not ask her any more till they got to her door, mostly because it was too loud to talk in the stairwell, and he could not afford the divided attention to keep his footing on the rickety steps. When she turned the key, entered, then shut the door and locked it behind them, he noted the sturdiness of the door—nearly all the clamour was silenced instantly as it slammed shut. The room was a suite, with sliding doors dividing two main rooms, the first in total darkness, the further one dark, too, but illumined by a red-glass-shaded lamp with the frame of a spider's web on a far end table. From the inner room there was a Victrola phonograph softly playing "Mad Mama's Blues," a rousing, gaily phrased song in English of dynamite and gunpowder and murdering everyone the singer Josie Miles sees, a singsong jazzy combo coming in scratchy behind her.

"Are you there, darling?" called a voice from the shadows of the further chamber, a tired voice, a young voice, a woman's.

"Yes, love," said Katharina, "but I'm not alone."

"Who's with you?"

"Just a fellow from the demonstration. Why don't you come and greet him?"

The sigh that followed was almost fierce.

"No, not *now*," the voice said, softer now, almost inaudible.

Katharina turned conspiratorially to Theodor then, and whispered, "I think Johanna's still recovering from last night. It was . . . quite a night."

She pulled the double doors shut, then flicked on a light, showing a parlour of sickly splendour. The wallpaper was brown and faded floral patterns, spotted here and there with something black and oily, the furniture spare and old. There was a small, high round table of chipped cherry-wood on which sat a tasselled drawstring lamp, prettily fin-de-siecle, and a large ashtray overflowing with cigarette butts and other, more exotic smoking fragments, spilling over onto a few magazines, *Der Sturm, Der Strom,* and something advertising itself as a "militant prostitute's weekly" from Hamburg called *Der Pranger.* Open beside these magazines, dusty with ashes and hanging a little precariously by the edge of the table, was an advanced-copy of a book featuring darkly-lit, orgiastic scenes of naked dancers of various genders and ages; it fell off the table as Theodor gazed into it like a slap—a somewhat startling thing that caused him to wince. Katharina just laughed, and picked the book up, closing it and tossing it back amidst the ashes. Theodor read the plain cover, the lurid images stolen from his view, the title *Magic: History, Theory, and Practice,* by a fellow named Ernst Schertel; then, shyly, he looked away. A long, low vermilion couch of vaguely oriental flavour was tucked into a corner, some bookcases on either side of it, and three mismatched, roughly-upholstered chairs huddled between it and the table. There was a window, but the heavy, oil-stained purple curtains were drawn, as the adjoining room's were, leaving it a completely open question whether it was midday or midnight.

The one thing that brightened the place, though in its aspect also darkened it rather, were a host of collages and photomontages, all modern, very recent or just a few years old, mostly clipped from magazines or ripped off lampposts and billboard hoardings, making a motley and a little disturbing collection of images. There were bits of machinery spliced onto women's body parts, parodies of Agitprop and the new Socialist Realism, and newspaper clippings of demonstrations, riots, and the forward march of Fascists. The clippings were easily of half a dozen languages and more than a dozen countries, of which Theo, who could reckon Russian fairly well, and Polish and English brokenly, could recognize the main issues: here a bit about the fight of Nestor Makhno and his free peasant army against the White and Red Armies in the Ukraine; there, a call for action in London, Paris, New York, Chicago, Toronto, San Francisco and Mexico City to protest the continued incarceration of Sacco and Vanzetti. A lot of these articles were ripped out of newspapers rather hastily, unintentionally all but ruined. There were also things that seemed *intentionally* ruined: A blue worker's uniform shirt stencilled with Cyrillic letters "Blue Blouse Theatre Troupe #1," with words scrawled in grease paint near the shredded hem—*Comrade Yuzhanin sure dresses us funny, don't he?* Assembled together beside it were pieces of a lithograph, ink-stained and rusted with several key shards missing, of what appeared a grotesque Prussian man in a top hat munching on a sandwich of skulls and spiked infantry helmets, and the words "God With Us"—looking as if it had been saved from a dustbin.

Beside these, there were a host of colourful playbills from events held in places like "Cabaret Voltaire" and "Galerie Dada" with Zurich addresses dated several years before, as well as a "farewell show" for some place here in Berlin called the "Galarie Der Sturm," dated earlier this year. A few posters from recent cinema-flicks hung here and there, including one for *Das Blut der Schwester,* with the same name cited as the flick's writer as the author of the book on the table beneath all the ashes, Ernst Schertel (whom, when Theodor asked about it, Katharina said was a theorist of naked dance, magic, and sadomasochism—a boy older than that clown Erik Boom!, yet a boy she also was "in *love* with"; the book on the table wouldn't be out till next year, but she was acquainted with the writer, even if not, to her regret, *intimately* so—at least, not *yet*). There were photos of many naked dancers here and there on the walls, too (now that the subject had come up). A dim snapshot from a Brownie camera showed what appeared a naked Celly de Rheidt doing that dance that got her into such trouble a couple years back—as a defrocked nun dancing with another naked woman meant to be the Virgin Mary. There was also an autographed photo of Anita Berber—the notorious drug-and-sex-fiend that had been in the papers a lot lately; the scrawled signature included some very rude words, insults really, that Katharina had evidently "earned" one lucky, drunken cabaret night, along with some lovely bruises. Other dancers Theodor didn't recognize were featured in other photos, mostly dressed scantily or not at all. One woman's outfit clothed but half her body—her left arm and leg—and hearkened to Ancient Egypt; her legs were shackled together by a rather short chain. Two theatre tickets were tacked not far from the photos, English words of a performance dated 1917, the title of which Theodor made out as "Spring Awakening," by a playwright with the German-sounding name of Frank Wedekind. Beside these was another snapshot, of what must have been Katharina at fifteen or sixteen with an old woman, arm-in-arm, both dressed smartly and modernly, in front of what Katharina told him was a New York theatre. Not far from that photo were a spread of pin-ups of various naked women, some of a lilting, Oriental flavour reminiscent of Theda Bara's films—an entirely different aesthetic than "normally" beautiful, *naturlich* German women, something deliberately strange, even perverse— with the magazine title *Die Freundin* printed above them all. An old poetry book featuring a cherub with a spear and a cat o' nine-tails and the words *Confirmo te Chrysmate* by a poet called *Dolorosa* nestled amidst these, nailed harshly and cruelly to the wall, the threaded booklet inviting any and all to partake of what lay within— the dog-eared pages seeming to have shared itself with many, tears, folds, mutilations, fiercest scribbles and rude doodles in the margins telling the tale of hundreds of hands' violations of the text. Beside this old book hung some pages torn out of a much newer-looking poetry book (but just as abused), called *Dances of Vice, Horror, and Ecstasy,* a collaboration of the notorious naked dancer who had so spat upon the grateful face of this girl taking off her ermine wrap and cloche before Theodor now and the dancer's partner, the nefarious Sebastian Droste. Plastered onto the wall at a little distance from these was a very well-preserved cover from some periodical declaring "Everyman His Own Football," featuring a spread of pictures of famous old German politicians, bearded and moustachioed and monocled, with the question **"Which one is prettiest?"**

Theodor wondered at it all, and found himself approving of the dark ambiance, all this weird art on these soiled walls, though he only partially knew why. He particularly liked a collage, or montage (he was shaky on the correct terms for such things) featuring the face of Frederick the Great, as played by the actor Otto Gebuhr in a recent cinema-flick, cut into very thin, jagged strips, in between which were scenes of dens of prostitutes, opium-addicts, and homosexuals of various genders in various suggestive poses, from some of the recent "asphalt" films that delved into such things. Exactly what was meant by the piece was unclear to Theodor (Katharina herself said the piece was done by a friend of hers, no one particularly "famous," and that she also did not know what the girl had "meant"). But Theodor liked looking at that icon of "proper" conservative, "heroic" Deutschland being *ripped apart*— quite *literally*—in such a way.

Katharina unlaced, then kicked off her calf-boots, setting them down against the wall by the tiny bathroom, beside another set of boots of the same poisonous green, but of a larger size. Beside these were an array of boots of her size as well as the latter's, black, brown, lacquered gold, cobalt blue, and several varieties of red. The laces, too, were different in each, black, white, maroon, and gold— though the style of them, sleek, unadorned leather of higher-than-average quality and higher-than-average heels—were the same—an almost uniform effect. Katharina took off Theodor's boots, too, kneeling before him as he scrambled, half-standing, half-leaning on the oily wall to help her. She set them a little apart from the others, and Theodor noted with the slightest shame their rough and dirty appearance next to the elegant, shiny fare beside them.

Katharina smiled up to him, then, from where she knelt by the boots. She gazed at him a moment, then arose slowly, gracefully, her eyes coyly fixed in his, and sat down on one of the armchairs, leaving Theodor with the choice of which of the others to collapse into. He chose the chair further from her.

"Johanna is who, now?" he asked.

"Someone I met. A good, good friend. She drinks a bit, but then, we all have our little vices. I'm afraid she won't really be ready to meet you for a few more hours at least."

"That's okay." Then, smiling, he ventured, "A friend of yours from the bar?"

Katharina laughed lightly.

"If you like," she said, intentionally vague. Then she laughed again. "I meet a lot of gals at that bar, liebling. Sometimes, they end up living with me, for a time. You wouldn't know it from how it is now, all quiet and afternoonlike, but this place can get to be quite the zoo sometimes."

"Other people live here, too?"

"Sometimes. Sometimes not. But I like it best when there's a crowd about. It helps me . . . well, it *helps* me. Helps me get outta my brain. You know?"

Theodor nodded.

"Still," she continued, "it's good to get time alone, too. Do you live with people, Theodor?"

"Just my Papa. He's disabled, and so I help him, you know, get around. He would've been at the demonstration today, if he didn't have his bad foot. Can't really stand, or march, any more. But in the old days, he went to a lot of things. He's an old Social Democrat, from way back in the day, when it was still banned, y'know, under Bismark."

"He's old, then?"

"Pretty. Mama left him, and took my older sister with. So, it's just him and me."

"You get along with him?"

Theodor smiled. Talking about his family was not something he usually did with strangers, and this girl was yet a stranger. But, he trusted her somehow, and told her candidly that the old man had been a bear to him when he was younger, and he still had a little resentment towards him; but, now, just lately, things had been better. Even though the father could not countenance, nor even try to understand what Theodor was doing with his life. The Social Democracy was more than, and less than, the good old Revolution. It had a respectability now, as it had aged, and Theodor's father had aged with it. It seemed to him a foolish thing, this Spartakist thing, something so wrong-headed the father could no longer talk about it.

"He's spent all his ire, venting his spleen, till there's nothing left in it to vent at me any more. I've been in the Spartakusbund almost since the Revolution—joined up in '19, when the ink in Versailles was still wet on the paper—and I've been dealing with all the things he would've warned me about for long enough that he's stopped bothering with his warnings. What can I say? He's the Old Deutschland, in many, many ways."

Katharina smiled coyly.

"Are you the New Deutschland, Theo?"

Theodor laughed, realizing he had the opportunity now to be quite pretentious, if he chose to be. He also chuckled at her shortening of his name, which in nineteen years he hadn't thought to do. Rather than answering the loaded question, he laughed, till she laughed with him, and he pursued the subject of family in order to change it.

"So," he said, "you have a Mama and a Papa, too?"

She smiled, squinting at him.

"If I told you I just sprouted from the earth, would you believe me?"

"Oh, no. The ocean is where I'd picture you coming from. Rising from it on a half-shell."

"Well, that makes sense. My family *is* in shipping."

"Shipping?"

"Yeah. They have something to do with ships, and carrying things in ships, and I don't really know what exactly they do with all the ships and the things in the ships, but I know it's made them a lot of money."

Theodor regarded her in an interested silence. So, she was bourgeois, then? That seemed a strange background for a girl with pink hair, a girl who mulled about in anarchist circles and went to demonstrations, a girl who lived in a place like this. She chuckled, shaking her head so her upturned curls shook with her. She anticipated his thoughts.

"Yeah, suβe," she chuckled, "my people are on the *other side* of things. That used to bug me, till I realized I'd done nothing to deserve it. And, like it or not, I can't change it either. Know what I mean?"

Theodor nodded.

"Yeah," he said. "I think this system's bad for all the classes, eventually. Nobody, on any side, is really all that happy. . . . Tell me the truth: you don't really get on with the old folks, do ya?"

"Well, Theo, if you owned a shipping line, a line that bought its steel from war machine conglomerates and used it to do what your government friends told you to do, putting down strikes and breaking up unions of shipwrights and sailors and dockers and stevedores, as your friends advise—to keep your money, which you love more than anything else—would you really want a daughter like me?"

Evidently, Katharina did not have the same compunctions about sharing her family strife with strangers as he. And, maybe her willingness to share her turmoil and his hesitancy to share his came from the same source: *class.* She did not want to be part of her background, whilst Theodor did. So, she freely discussed her angers, as he hid his, out of respect for the same class struggle, and the need to align oneself properly. This, at least, was what Theodor concluded then.

Theodor decided he liked Katharina; and Katharina had already decided she liked him. They spoke freely of the class system, the ambiguities as well as what was obvious and clear, for the next quarter hour. Katharina's family was not just a wealthy family; it was also a Jewish family, one relatively new to money. It was strange, she said, being from somewhere where you both oppressed and yet suffered discrimination. Theodor understood. He had a great love of Jewish culture and Jewish people. His father's best friend, a tradesman and one-time activist in the Jewish Labour Bund, whom Theodor was taught to call "uncle" from the earliest ages, had been knifed in a bar fight with fascists just last year, all because he "looked the part" of a Jew too well for their liking. Jewish thinkers had been crucial in the development of Marxism, starting with Marx himself, extending all the way to martyred Red Rosa, who had led the faction he'd pledged his life to. Rich people were, of course, rich people, and Theodor understood Katharina's condemning of her family. But hate was hate, and he was more than familiar with the false linking of being rich and being Jewish, as if one was the other, and he hated the people who were making that link.

They talked a little about that, too, and Katharina and Theodor warmed to each other even more, as Katharina got up and offered them both some fine cherry schnapps from a well-stocked cabinet. Theodor gratefully accepted the drink, and he got up to sit down in the chair nearer her.

Johanna arose over the next hours, and opened the suite doors to let in her room-mate and her room-mate's friend, apologizing for her unsavoury attitude earlier. Theodor had no ill feelings, indeed had noticed no such "unsavouriness," as she said, but Johanna apologized yet again. She was a tall woman, thickly, lusciously built, and very pale, with black and unfashionably long hair, which she let hang down. Her dress was not conservative in the least, however. She was wearing a black and silken thing laced in gold and scarlet, a kimono, which would be barely legal outside this room, something she'd evidently slept in the night before. Theodor felt a little awkward, addressing this woman, a stranger, so scantily attired, out of a sense of propriety that was more shyness. But the lady Johanna had no shame about it at all, and he soon settled down on a love seat with Katharina girlishly sitting down by his feet, leaning her head on his lap, as Johanna sat on an old bare-wood Shaker rocker spangled with embroidered pillows, her beautiful pallid legs stretched over a plush, vermilion ottoman, incongruously paired with it.

She treated Theodor as if he were the most interesting boy she'd ever met; she had that charm. Katharina told him later that she made her living as a prostitute, a high class courtesan, and that she'd done "interesting things" with high-powered businessmen clients and even heads of state. She proceeded, and had long done so, as an independent woman, working away from the brothels of the Alex and the West End, eschewing madams and pimps, her anarchism showing in her decision to refuse the *Reglementierung* demanding she register with the government to ply her trade. She spat on the restrictions of the reglementierung, the proscriptions on where to live, and how to live, the mandatory health inspections by the quacks she spat were nought but "pussy-pressers," the monthly interviews with cops from a division of the police force just for "Kontroll-Girls," as the legal, regulated prostitutes were called. Johanna was a free woman, and she'd rather die than give any token of her freedom to bureaucrats and policemen who existed only for the consternation of the free.

She smiled at Theodor, laughing at his awkward jokes, making him feel well at ease in the unfamiliar place, as if she'd long known the arts of making men feel at ease. But she didn't really like men at all, their state, their bodies, their very spirit in the Fatherland. It was all a show, Katharina later said; but Theodor could never tell what the show was for, nor what Johanna could ever gain by putting it on for such an obviously poor and powerless boy like him. Katharina would explain that Johanna's moods were as volatile as the weather, and that, if he hung around, he would see them change many times. Johanna might even turn her ire on him, though she did not yet know him well. Most of it had to do with how much she'd had to drink.

At the moment, though, they were not drinking. They were smoking, rather, French cigarettes dipped in opium. Theodor had never indulged in this before, and was quite bowled over with the feeling. Katharina and Johanna had more experience in this realm, and as Theodor lazed on the love seat, they began to dance a queer dance in front of him.

It was a queer dance, intimate and slow, with no music on the phonograph, though Theodor swore he could hear some, distantly in the background; the jazz combo in the flat below, perhaps. Amidst this serenade, hinting just beyond the periphery, was the cackling of that nameless old man in some flat further below, laughing and laughing, little queer chromatic wisps amidst the violins and the coronets. The two women spun and twirled, then mimsily flailed, as two willow trees in a midnight summer breeze. Then, a look came into Johanna's eyes, a look of almost anger, but cooler, and more severe. Katharina evidently recognized that look, for at once her face became one of silent, fawning awe, her grey-blue eyes big and open, her smile gone.

Johanna turned abruptly, and returned to her chair, stretching her legs on the ottoman again, her face turned away to the wall, to a large, silver-framed mirror in which long-extinct butterflies were pressed. Katharina fell to her knees, and crawled over to where her lover sat. Then, with her eyes big and plaintive, she whispered something Theodor could not hear.

Johanna regarded her with the same severe countenance, and lifted her hand, just a little, off the armrest. Katharina instantly kissed it. She took it in her hands as if she were a pilgrim in a medieval cloister, allowed by a high church cardinal to kiss the holiest relic of a cathedral she'd spent half a lifetime wending toward. She kissed and kissed, with a little girl's affection, even a puppy's, till abruptly Johanna pulled away and slapped her, the crack hard enough to hear across the room. Then Johanna turned away again, toward the wall.

Not deterred by this, Katharina crawled on her hands and knees to the ottoman, brushing the ends of her hair on the woman's feet in a way that reminded Theodor of Mary Magdalene, washing the feet of Christ, and whispered her sweet entreaty again. This time Theodor caught the words *"meine Domina, meine Göttin, sehr schöne, sehr stark . . ."* repeated over and over again like a mantra. Johanna looked down at her with an austere expression, and with the slightest nod, granted the favour her lover begged. *"Sie können,"* she breathed, *"Sie **müssen**."* She wiggled her toes, and Katharina bent to kiss them, opening her mouth a little bit, then wider, to taste every curve of Johanna's sculpted, long, high-arching feet. This went on for more than a quarter hour, Johanna stretching luxuriously in her heavily-cushioned chair, Katharina doing homage to her, knees bruising on the thinly carpeted hardwood floor, both seeming to find fulfilment in the degradation. After a long while of this, Johanna snapped her fingers, and her slave pulled away, as if the shapely toes and heels she worshipped had just shocked her with electricity. She knelt there, her face open, awaiting some order from her mistress, who at length lilted her desire.

"I *thirst*," she groaned prettily, closing her eyes and turning again toward the wall and the mirror. As if on cue, Katharina crawled clear across the room, ascending only slightly to find the mix of liqueurs on the mantle beside the great canopy bed that was her mistress' desire. Then, walking over on tiptoe, she knelt before Johanna, and offered up the glass with a bowed head.

Johanna accepted the drink, sipped it, then spat it into Katharina's face with an indignant grunt.

"You mixed it very *poorly*," she rasped, "very, *very* poorly. Drink it—instantly!—and tell me how you meant me to stomach it!"

Katharina gulped the whole mixture down till she choked, her face pained and sickened.

"I'm sorry, mistress," she whimpered. "I'll—I'll try again."

"Less champagne," Johanna commanded coldly, "and more Vana Tallinn. Any *fool* would know that."

"Yes, mistress. Forgive me."

"Just mix another—at once!"

Katharina did mix another, and again offered it to Johanna, who this time was satisfied. She reached down, and stroked Katharina's pinkish hair with a loving affection, the first affection she'd shown her in all the ritual.

"That's it," she smiled to her. "Now, *meine lieblich sklavin—come to me . . .*"

Johanna opened her legs, so long, so luscious and beautiful, and lifted her kimono flap, in such a way as to hide her delicately-haired sex from Theodor, but enough for Katharina to view it. Katharina smiled in utter exhilaration, and instantly bent down to immerse herself in it. She kissed her mistress' sex for a long, long moment, enveloping her whole face in it, and Theodor realized even with the sleepy opium that he was being let into a profound intimacy. But Johanna and Katharina proceeded as if he weren't even there, they alone in the room, hidden in the shadow and the night. From time to time, Johanna pulled Katharina by her hair, jerking her up to gaze into her imperious eyes for minutes on end. They said things then in whispers, their exchanges lost on Theodor; but then, she would push her back, and allow her (or, *force* her, choking and writhing) to continue her homage.

It was hours, it seemed, till they were done with their ritual,

Johanna moving her long foot under Katharina's skirt, forcing her slavegirl's legs wide against the tight skirt, massaging her secret places with a precision and skill that made her slave gasp and sigh in exultation, her groans muffled in Johanna's sex as her mistress forced her head to remain there. Johanna, though her eyes glazed over for the briefest instant, made no sound. Theodor nodded off for a time, and when he regained consciousness, the two were talking and joking in a friendly, easy and equal manner, their clothing unruffled, no sign between them of anything out of the ordinary, to the point where Theodor debated with himself whether he'd really witnessed it at all, or if it were all just an opium dream. It wasn't until much later, round midnight, when a group of young anarchists and artists and what seemed perennially down-and-out types, long used to living on the fringes, had come to fill the rooms with jovial laughter and playfully fierce debate, that Katharina made reference to it all.

Johanna had gone out for the night, and they sat in a dark corner in the parlour, on the oriental divan, as the young men and women, and a scattering of older ones, danced and drank and smoked things in the chambers with an unfettered abandon, sipping from common bottles and trading various pills like candy. Katharina smiled to Theodor, curling into his arm, and said, "I hope you didn't mind."

"Mind? Mind what?"

"Johanna and me. Earlier."

Theodor regarded her drunkenly, curiously in the haze.

"Of course not," he said. "I'm—I'm kinda honoured, actually."

Katharina smiled, and pecked him on the cheek.

"She doesn't generally like an audience," she explained, "but, somehow, she knew you might be the kind of fellow who wouldn't mind. Besides, she could tell I liked you."

"Really?"

"Sure. In fact, I was quite surprised she didn't order me to give you a blow job—or at least rub your feet."

Theodor had come with Katharina, earlier in the day, thinking on his attraction to her, wondering if there was a chance it could be mutual. But this openness was more than he'd hoped for. He honestly wouldn't know what he would have done, he said, if this stranger had been ordered by another stranger to do things with him, for him, after the opium and the dancing. But, he said, it was nice to get it all out in the open.

"Yes, it is," Katharina smiled to him. "Tell me, Theodor—can you stay the night?"

Theodor sighed hard.

"God, I'd love to," he said. "God! I'd love to!"

"But, you can't?"

"No."

"Why not?"

"Because o' my Papa. And, the Party. I've got to leaflet outside the factories tomorrow, early, before dawn, to catch the morning shift. And my Papa gets a little surly if I stay out without telling him about it."

"Well, call him! We've got a phone."

"Yeah, but we don't."

Katharina sighed, and pulled away.

"A pity," she said. "I really wanted to fuck you, baby."

Theodor smiled, a little surprised, but not put off, by the honesty.

"Well, if I was put on the spot, I'd hafta say I wouldn't mind that either, sister. Is it possible to—to get a rain check on that?"

"Of course! When ya wanna get together again?"

"Well, I'm off work after Friday. Maybe you'd like to meet me after work that night?"

"Where d'you work?"

"At a warehouse, down by the docks on the east harbour. It's decent money, and the union's strong. I've got a lotta comrades there. I'd love ya to meet 'em. And then, you know, we could grab somethin' to eat."

"Sounds good, man. Write down your address, both the warehouse and your flat. I'll visit you soon. Until then—*c'mere!*"

She pulled him toward her, and kissed him fully on the lips. He kissed her back, and for a brief moment, he didn't think of his father, or the Party, or his job, or anything else. For a moment, he thought he'd turn his back on all his obligations—for the first time in his life. But then, he recovered himself, and ended the kiss, promising to see her again soon. She walked him down the steps, into the street, and waited with him for a tram. They kissed once more, and then he was gone.

"Who was the boy?" asked her comrade knowingly when Katharina returned to the apartment. She took a drink of the bottle she offered, and said, "A Spartakist."

     "A commie?"

     "Yeah."

     "What are you doin' with a commie, man?"

     Katharina smiled.

     "Nothin'," she said, "*yet* . . ."

Chapter 2

When Theodor stumbled in around half past one, his father was waiting.

"And where the hell have you been?"

Theodor regarded his father in a dizzy, sourly sobering state. He'd been feeling pretty good, thinking on the anarchist girl, and his good fortune at having bumped into her. He did not want to end this feeling with the inevitable confrontation with his Papa. But, he loved his old man, too, and felt a wave of guilt now for not having been there to fix him his dinner, get him his pilsner, change the dressings on his foot. He smiled.

"Met somebody at the demonstration, Vati," he said.

"What?"

"I met somebody at the demonstration."

"What? Another one o' your communist friends?"

"No. An anarchist, actually."

The old man groaned. His face was exactly like Theodor's, just aged forty years. His eyes were dark, an almost onyx, his skin quite pale in contrast, and his chin came to a sharp point, exactly as Theodor's. What hair there was left on him was remarkably unwhitened by the times he'd lived, a few silver flecks in a slick of black. The old man's hair had darkened rather than lightened over his years, much as Theodor's, who had been a toe-headed baby and was now at nineteen sandy-blonde, sliding toward sandy-brown; if Theodor made it to sixty, his hair would likely be as black as his father's. The old man's belly was big and pronounced over his belt, his arms and frame that of a boxer, aged a generation past his prime. Laugh lines in his face told the story of smiles he'd carried since the nineteenth century, though they told the story of many frowns also. His nose was bulbous and Roman, a little crooked, as if he'd blocked his share of punches with it in his time. This nose was the only feature of his face that didn't resemble his son's; his son had the small, Belgian nose of his mother. The old man was dressed in a sleeveless under-shirt and ragged, stained pyjama pants, and had his bad foot up on a chair, under the table, his cane resting against his side.

"I'm sorry," Theodor said, "that I'm so late."

"What do I care?" the father said. "You're old enough now, to do as you like."

The sting of baiting his guilt was worse than a blow would

have been. Theodor sighed. He would not dignify this attempt on his conscience with a response.

"It was a good demonstration, Vati," he said. "Too bad you couldn't get there."

"Yeah, too bad. . . . I heard there were arrests."

"Yeah."

"You know, you could get yourself into trouble, son. I know I've told ya that a lot in the past few years—but, it's still true."

"Vati, as long as there's capitalists, there'll be trouble."

The old man looked down, and nodded slowly to himself, smiling a little.

"You sound like a young Wilhelm Liebknecht."

"You know, his son, Karl, was quite a speaker, too."

"Yeah . . ."

The old man looked down at his belly, and fed himself another of the many pilsners that had made that belly. He sat at their little table in their little kitchen, which with the bedroom and the bath was the only place in the world that was theirs. The kitchen was bright, despite the low illumination, owing to the bright yellow wallpaper, which featured sharply red flowers in columns, from ceiling to floor. The icebox hummed in its place by the little stove, all greasy and brown over the white. A little mouse was poking around in the corner; in the silence, it pattered its way back into the wainscoting, and disappeared.

"It keeps me company," the father said of the mouse, looking at it leave the room through its hole.

Theodor was so angry, so guilty, that he left the room, going into their shared bedchamber, all without telling his father of the girl he'd met, something which, even if she was an anarchist, even if she did dress like a slut, even if she did have pink hair, would have tickled the old man, and led him to shed this passive-aggressive manner in which he treated Theodor. No, Theodor didn't bother telling him about it. Why bother?

His father was dying. A combination of tuberculosis, slowly eating away at his leg, and another, vaguer thing, but much, much grimmer: a cancer, which the doctors said was slow-acting but sure. It would kill him some year, this year, next year, perhaps, if lucky, the year after that. But it was sure to overwhelm him in the end, just as the Roman army overwhelmed Spartacus and his slave rebellion, so long ago.

The father did not think on his own death. His mind was on his son, always. He drank, and he wondered, a creeping certainty. The father looked at the wainscoting, in the harsh light of the overhead bulb, swinging on the fraying wire like a noose in the shadow, and concluded his son was going to die.

Chapter 3

Katharina came to meet Theodor that Friday, at the end of his shift in the warehouse near the docks where he worked. His workday had not been pleasant. The place was a stronghold of the SPD, and like most in that reactionary, once-socialist party, the workers there were a lot less idealistic about Left unity than was the young Theodor. He had to fight the urge to condemn the lot of them; if it weren't for his father, whom he loved (and who still voted SPD, despite their past betrayals), and his uncle and all the others of that generation he'd known and loved, Theodor might well reason all the workers who supported the Social Democrats were miserable, unreachable thugs. Some of them had lain for him in a corner of the warehouse, where they'd tried to intimidate him. They'd not chosen his KPD membership as their sticking point, however.

"Hey, Priser!" they taunted him. "How come we never see ya with a girl?"

Theodor just looked at them, five of them, all bigger than he.

"You like boys, Priser, don't ya?" they jeered.

"What the hell's it to ya?!" he spat back.

One of the fellas looked to the others and laughed, "He *admits* it, then!"

"You know what your problem is?" Theodor taunted back. "You're a bunch of backward lackeys! You know that? You'd rather pick on one o' yer own than do a goddamn thing to liberate yourselves! I *do* like girls—but, if you wanna label me—I'd take *hot-brother fairy-boy* over *dumb-ox capitalist boot-licker* any day!"

The fellas did not like this, not at all. They stopped their laughing and their taunting, and looked like they meant to *do* something to the young Communist. But then, a couple other fellas came, comrades of Theodor, and told the bastards to move on— unless they wanted a real fight right there on the floor. These, but three of them, all had long bits of metal or wood in their hands, and did not seem at all afraid to use them.

"Fuck it," the first group dismissed, and dispersed, cursing the Spartakists in general and Theodor in particular. Theodor turned to his comrades and thanked them.

"No problem, brother," said one of them, an older man, almost of Theodor's father's generation, a fellow named Maximilian. Old Max, he was called, short and wide-shouldered, with salt-and-pepper hair, black eyes, and a grizzled moustache. He clapped Theodor on the back.

"Get home, comrade," he said, and the others, all between his age and Theodor's, told him the same.

Nothing more came of it, till the very end of the shift some minutes later, when Theodor got his time-card punched, and made for the doors. His tormentors, minus one, were waiting for him there.

"Your faggot comrades ain't here to protect ya now, eh Priser?" they taunted.

That's when Katharina appeared.

"Hey there, baby!" she said, running to hug him. Theodor was happy to see her, and ignored the ugly men in the threshold of the warehouse.

"Hey, schätzelein," he smiled, hugging her back.

"How you been?" she asked.

"Well, been better, but—"

"Hey, lady!" called the phalanx from the door frame. "You know your boyfriend's a cocksucker, right?"

Theodor was mortified. But, without batting an eye, without even turning her head to regard them, Katharina just laughed and shouted—"Yeah! I know! He sucks my cock every night!"

"I'm pretty fuckin' good at it, too!" Theodor laughed in step. "Ain't I, sister?"

"I got no complaints!" she laughed.

The bully boys were nonplussed at this solidarity. Defeated, they shouted at their heels—"Go on—give each other syphilis, then! A slut and a faggot! What a *happy couple!*"

Katharina was bewildered, and getting riled.

"What kinda arschlochs do you work with?!" she shouted, this time turning her head (they were a good ways away now, heading down a service road between the buildings).

Theodor laughed evilly.

"Social Democrats!" he spat, even louder than she.

Katharina laughed, throwing her head back.

"Does a Party proud!" she chuckled viciously. The bullies shouted more shit at them, but by then they were out of earshot.

They walked a while, through the depressed, darkened district, deciding to get a bite at a little place Theodor knew. It was a sad little cafeteria, very small, and at that moment, very empty.

Most of the later shifts frequented the larger cafeterias, closer to the warehouse district, or the beer halls further on. Theodor liked this place because it was rarely too crowded, even at times that were peak times at places just blocks away. He figured the place was owned somewhat dubiously, a kind of grey market enterprise, veering toward the black, a front for the contraceptives and other contraband the owner ran out of the back.

Theodor offered to pay for their meal there, but Katharina would have none of it. Indeed, *she* offered to pay, which surprised Theodor in a pleasant way. He got a meal of grilled Thuringer and sauerkraut, a creamy potato salad with pickles and radishes, and a glass of beer. Katharina matched his beer, but just got some sauerkraut and the salad, and informed him that she was a vegetarian.

"Really?" he said, sitting down in a little booth across from her.

"Yeah, for a little over a year, now."

"Why?"

"It's just part of my anarchy, liebling. I don't wanna oppress people, as far as I can help it. And animals are people, too."

"It's probably healthier, too, I suppose."

"Sure. But, that's not why I do it, really."

"Huh. Well, I hope you don't mind if *I* stay a carnivore."

"I don't believe in imposing my will on people. I think that's my main difference with you commies. You guys *do* impose."

This caught Theodor off guard.

"Yeah," he said. "I'd say we do. But, if you're up against people who are doin' that, too, what choice do ya have?"

"Dialectics, I suppose."

"That's right."

They sat a moment in silence. It was an uncomfortable silence, in which both reflected on a point they'd not acknowledged before: they were different. Of course, they *knew* they were different, in their way, and had known it since they'd first met. But, here, the difference seemed to have the seeds of becoming a *conflict*, and neither knew what to do with that. Both had been schooled to despise the other's politics, even though neither really knew much about what the other believed. "Dialectics" was something Katharina had said in a tongue-in-cheek way, mocking the idea of it without really caring much about what it was. It was just something Marxists said, she thought, and they used the term to justify anything. Socialists all said that word, from Bernstein to Kautsky to Luxemburg, and the differing factions used that "logic" to come up with completely different, even opposing conclusions about the world. But, to Theodor, the word *meant* something. It meant nothing less than the basis for his whole world-view. And, in that embarrassed silence, each knew the other's view on that (and, by implication, much, much more) was completely antithetical to their own.

Katharina laughed, bringing them out of their discomfort by inquiring what those "Social Democrats" meant by their jeering of him.

"You work with arschlochs," she laughed. "What the hell was all that about?"

Theodor smiled.

"I don't really know. Those guys don't like me much."

"So, they called you a cocksucker just 'cause they don't like you?"

"Basically. But, I guess—I guess they've got their reasons."

"*Are* you a cocksucker?"

Theodor looked at her oddly. She was direct, and shameless. But, while this was a little discomforting, it was also the reason he was beginning to be crazy about her. She shared everything, and expected you to do the same. Very well, then . . .

"Would it bother you if I was?" he said, just as directly, looking her dead in the eye.

She smiled, undaunted.

"Actually," she said, "it'd probably turn me on."

"Really?"

"Oh, yeah! You already know I like girls. It'd tickle me to no end if you liked boys, too."

Theodor looked down at his sausage and smiled reflectively. He was being offered, he realized, a freedom he'd never been allowed before. All his private thoughts, all his secret fears, could at this moment cease to be so private, so secret. Yes, as a matter of fact, he'd entertained the thought of being with men. Just, he'd never admitted it to anyone—not even himself, really. But, now?

Now . . .

"I've never really told anybody about this," he said, "but, I've had dreams. Dreams of . . . well . . ."

"Sleeping with men?"

Theodor sighed. This was it. He'd had dreams like that since puberty. Not *a lot*, but enough. He'd never told a living soul. And, he'd never acted on any of it. Since he was thirteen, he'd been torn between feelings of disgust, attraction, and indifference toward these dreams, each coming in its turn. His own amorous experience was not very extensive. He'd had but two girlfriends in all that time, one a slight, dark-featured girl who had done little more with him than kiss, and another girl, blonde and voluptuous, who had done everything *but* sleep with him (depending on how one defined "sleeping" with). He'd learnt a little about it all, enough to know he liked it. But, he thought, there was so much more to know.

"Of course there is," she agreed, very seriously, almost solemnly. "I've been influenced a lot by what Magnus Hirschfeld has to say."

"I'm not sure I know the man."

"Really? Huh. Well, he's a famous sexologist—you know, somebody who studies sexuality in the modern world."

"You mean, like Freud and those psychologists study sex?"

"A *little* like Freud and them. But, where Freud talks about sexual variation simply *existing*, Hirschfeld and his comrades say the different variations should actually be *encouraged*. He's spoken all over the world, championing sexual freedom and the almost unlimited variation that exists in nature as our human rights. Hundreds, thousands—maybe *millions* of people have become liberated because of what he's said and written. The Institute for Sexual Science—right here in Berlin—is a fantastic, priceless library of sexological material, sexual philosophy and fiction and poetry and erotica. There's books there by Karl Heinrich Ulrichs— that great campaigner for queer rights in the last century—and also stuff by Iwan Bloch and Albert Eulenburg and other sexologists Magnus has worked with. And, too, there's D.H. Lawrence and E.M. Forster, Annie Besant and Anna Elisabet Weirauch—Radclyffe Hall, Grete von Urbanitzki, Ernst Schertel, Edward Carpenter—oh! hundreds and *hundreds* of great sexy writers, Theo! Have you ever read Edward Carpenter?"

"Why, no."

"He's an English writer—over seventy years old, now— and still goin' strong! He goes even further than Hirschfeld and the sexologists, I think, even though he's from the older generation. I've got books by him like *Civilisation, Its Cause and Cure, The*

Intermediate Sex, and a great feminist work he wrote years ago called *Love's Coming-of-Age*. He calls himself a 'mystical socialist'—he believes civilisation isn't some great achievement, but is actually a *disease* human societies go through, a stage which never lasts more than a thousand years and is always built on oppression and unhealthiness."

"Didn't Freud write something like that? That civilisation causes neurosis? I heard somebody speaking on a street corner once, saying that."

"Freud *does* say that—you're right. But he concludes that that's just the way things are. We just can't do any better. Carpenter takes issue with it all—takes the bloody Minotaur by the horns and glares it in the eye—then rips its filthy head off! He doesn't say civilisation *causes* disease—he goes all the way and says civilisation *is the disease!"*

They laughed together at this, Katharina heartily, Theodor a trifle more tentatively. This was all new to him. He was not the heppest cat in the hep capitol—he was almost sheltered by some standards. Yet deep down, in the place where his darkest thoughts discoursed with one another, in conflicts he only became aware of when they arose into his dreams, he knew the heresies this pretty girl spoke of now were sure to find comrades and kin. She went on, eyeing him in a warmer way than before.

"Old Edward lives with a working class lover named George Merrill—they've lived together for years on a communal nudist farm in rural England—beautiful old daddies, both of them, Theo! I've corresponded with them, a little. But my great aunt—kind of the 'rebel matron' of my family—actually got to meet them, years ago. I still have a signed copy of *Love's Coming of Age* that she got on a visit to England before the war. Edward's written, and both his and George's lives have proven, that 'Eros is the great leveller'—queer love can transcend class and race, can destroy all the nonsensical hierarchy of our wretched, civilised culture. Queer love can bond people whom this world's hierarchies have long separated into this side and that—bourgeois and proletarian, Jew and Gentile, male and female—and all the rest of it. Eros is the only Deity I really acknowledge any more, Theo—the way all the fags and dykes write about it in *Die Freundschaft—Friendship,* a magazine I've been reading for years now, about queer spirituality and relationships. Ah, Eros, darling—the 'life-wish' of Freud, y'know?—the thing I have to make up my mind to embrace every day, waking up to the wretchedness of this world. Eros—the force that makes the blood burn red!—the thing that drives us to fuck like angelic, demonic beasts! Nothing can stand in its way, Theo. The bloody churches and the bloody governments have been trying to suppress it for thousands of years—but they can never quite stamp it out, can they? It'll overthrow all their bleeding empires one day, mein schätze. . . ."

She sighed, and laughed at herself. "It's all very freeing, Theo. Homosexuality, bisexuality, gender inversions, transvestitism, and all the dark, pretty 'perversities' people get into nowadays—fetishes, sadism, masochism, voyeurism, exhibition—a thousand-and-one unique and defiant lusts!—all these things have a *political* character. If we stand with Revolution, we've gotta be open to these things, too. A *sexual* revolution has to be part of any greater *social* revolution. D'you agree?"

Theodor nodded.

"So," she smiled, coyly, "d'you wanna sleep with men, or not?"

This brought the conversation back to its original drift, and Theodor realized he'd not answered her question. Could he now? *Should* he?

Why the hell not?

"Sure," he smiled. "I'd love to sleep with men. Why? Got any in mind?"

Katharina smiled coyly again, and said nothing for a moment, her beautiful blue-grey eyes studying him, as if making a calculation in her head.

"Yes," she said, clipped and certain. "Yes, Theo. I've got a lotta boys I know. We can arrange for you to lose that fag cherry, any time you want."

Theodor smiled, also coyly.

"I wouldn't mind losing my heterosexual cherry, either, you know."

She laughed out loud.

"*That,* liebling, can *also* be arranged . . ."

They went back to her place, to find a vibrant gathering of mostly younger people dancing and drinking. Theodor found them a queer mix of the gregarious and the hostile, as if a closed circle, used to persecution, therefore willing to throw the first blow rather than wait to be attacked. Yet, toward one another, there was something decidedly affectionate, even familial.   This was Katharina's family, more than any high-born blood tie she'd done her best to defy. Theodor sat comfortably among them, though he'd the odd feeling he was being allowed into some private, even secret place, some foreign enclave, as if he'd stepped from the busyness of modern Berlin into a medieval Gypsy encampment, or a Sufi hermitage in some hidden, moonlit desert of Araby.

Some older, frailly-built little Irish fellow in a beat-up fedora and rolled up sleeves on his pale, skeleton arms was playing a violin, something prettily Eastern, as the hubbub of the fifteen or twenty others squeezing into the corners of the little flat speaking in more than several tongues seemed unconscious lyrics to his folk song.   A tall, full-framed young American fellow was softly strumming a banjo in lazy accompaniment, a bottle of Clicquot Club ginger ale bubbling with bootleg Kentucky whiskey beside him. A woman with a small baby, dressed in motley rags, was breastfeeding the infant, rocking and bouncing it absently as someone handed her a marijuana cigarette, which she puffed and breathed its smoke into the mouth of another woman with short, oiled hair in a neck tie, who breathed it back in prelude to a kiss.   The mother's name was "Erika," a German name, though she looked to be a gypsy, her baby named "Chevali," which she said meant "girl" in the Romani tongue. The androgynous woman with the tie, a butch dandy of the "garçonne" style, was a person who had had several names in the course of the last few years, and now answered to a man's name Theo didn't quite catch.   A trio of travellers, evidently refugees from political tumult in Italy or Greece, snored pleasantly in a far corner, two of them cradling one another as if brothers (or perhaps something more intimate), the third cradling a small pistol. Four or five younger folks, informally studentish and of at least two genders, were gathered on and around the oriental divan, passing a jug of cheap wine among them, and composing a long, disjointed poem on a roll of toilet paper that just kept getting longer and longer as they took turns scribbling and sketching. Scattered here and there were decidedly more "serious-looking" types, the kind of sharp-eyed, stubble-faced, rail-like fellows you might imagine planting a bomb somewhere or making an impromptu, inciting speech on a street corner.   But there were at least as many clowns, as many pretty, low-rent dandies, as many persons of proudly dubious gender, and two or three toddlers with scarcely any clothes on running about. These people all knew Katharina, and knew her new fellow, the first by many a long late-night conversation and the sharing of the warmth of sex and drugs, the latter by rumour. Things remained pleasant for more than an hour before the first challenge was levelled at this stranger their Katharina had brought amongst them.

"So," the woman with the baby said sharply to Theodor, "you're a commie, then?"

"That's right," Theodor said, as ready to defend himself as he was to defend his views from the SPD bastards down at the warehouse.

"Why?" she pressed.

"Why not?"

"All governments are fucked, man," declared a tall, slight fellow with longish, raven hair and a little goatee and spectacles from the divan, in a Swiss accent. He wore simple, shabby clothes of browns and blacks, whose folds could not quite hide the compass round his neck, its needle wavering between a spread of magnets hanging loosely, randomly round it. "Your Russia is no more free than the bloody Czar was, you know."

"You been there, man?" Theodor challenged the strangely-clad fellow.

"No."

"Well, why pretend to be an expert on something you ain't never seen?"

"So, you're sayin' you *have* been there?"

"As a matter of fact, yeah, I have."

"And what did you find there, eh?"

Before Theodor could answer, Johanna had come into the room, dressed to kill, with a spread of undergarments, all black and red, with garter-belts keeping her lacy stockings upon her shapely legs, skimpy underwear that just teased at the revealing, and an elaborate corset which parodied the era they'd just left, the antebellum world of Victorian, Wilhelmine prudery. She twirled a riding crop in her hands.

"Who's been *naughty?*" she said, her eyes searching the room of anarchists sprawling on the floor in various knots. They all gazed up at her in wonder and laughter.

"*Theo* has!" giggled Katharina, playfully shoving his side.

"I dunno about *that,*" Theodor said, chuckling a little.

"Theo's a state socialist," Katharina explained. "A dictator of the proletariat."

"Oh, that's *very naughty*," Johanna said, in mock severity, and put her riding crop up to his chin, forcing his face up to hers.

"What *are* you going to *do* with this *naughty* communist?" Katharina giggled, and there were giggles from others round them. Theodor felt the joke, and played along. It diffused the situation entirely, leaving the young critics to go back to her baby and his poetry. In a moment, nobody could recall that there was some real, pressing issue of difference in politics between Theodor and the rest; all they could see was that the young, handsome (if conservatively dressed) fellow was involved with the reigning lady of their scene, the tender, playfully cruel dominatrix whom so many young women and men had aspired to playing with over the months and years they'd been a part of it.

Johanna's interest was only temporary, though, and entirely tongue-in-cheek. She was actually dressed up for a client, whom she awaited with a businesslike detachment. She would "punish" some bureaucrat tonight, for the awful crimes he'd committed in the era of the Kaiser. Theodor listened with guarded interest. Johanna seemed to take herself seriously, even though her tone was mocking. She really did have such a client, Katharina said, a regular, who was an old Prussian type with a shaved head, a handlebar moustache, even a monocle. By day, Katharina laughed, he was an important and thoroughly disgusting civil servant, responsible for the dole rosters of the unemployed. Theodor thought of his father, wasting away in their little hovel of a flat, and realized this bastard had power over him, and by association, much of the Berlin proletariat. And the old Prussian had a twinge of conscience about it all, evidently, for among his many fetishes was the trampling of important papers he would bring, lay at Johanna's feet, and cringe and cower as the whip-lady squashed his livelihood under her stiletto heels.

They did not wait for the client to appear, though, Katharina, Theodor, and her friends. Around midnight, the whole party save the sleeping Mediterranean trio emptied out of the place, and spilled onto the straβen, to wander toward the Tiergarten, where they would mingle with the homeless peasants who had come into the city to find work, and with them were a kind of underground culture there in the night. They sat with some of the young men on the bum, and exchanged cheap apple schnapps and angry words about the government and the rich, there on the park benches, in the shadows of the shanties that made a ramshackle village amidst the trees. There, under the stars, Katharina and Theodor kissed and fondled, becoming more prone on their park bench as the night waned on.

"Wanna do it here?" Katharina asked with a wicked smile.

"Here?" Theodor asked, hot but nervous. "In the park?"

"People fuck here all the time, Theo. Why not here?"

"I—I dunno. I mean, I *want* to. But, the Bullen—"

"Fuck 'em, man! C'mon—you want your first time to be memorable, eh? Well, it's *romantic*, here, under the stars. Y'know?"

And with the drunken sounds of wrangling youth, anarchist diatribes and dirty jokes, an old sailor's song with a rusty accordion somewhere distant, the sounds of the nightbirds and the traffic and the wind, Theodor decided to take up the offer.

He'd been a master of certain techniques, over his brief years of sexual life, becoming quite brilliant at tasting and pleasuring a woman with his tongue and fingers. His last lover, Gretchen, had craved his hot mouthing of her neck, breasts, and sex, as she'd given him an occasional taste of the reverse. But, fears of pregnancy, and a Catholic guilt that allowed her to break every taboo but one, had left them both still technical virgins, before she'd dropped him to go with a Brownshirt. Katharina had no such fears, no such guilt. She'd had an operation when she was thirteen that had sterilized her, a suggestion of the doctors that had been poking and prodding her since a babe, diagnosing her with all manner of diseases that she may or mayn't have had, her rich mother's projected hypochondria enfeebling her daughter from the earliest ages. She recalled the operation as a painful invasion, and proof, if ever she needed more, that her parents cared little or nought for her, leaving her brothers to carry on the family line. But Katharina laughed at it now. It allowed her to do things like this, all without worry, and so it was no bad thing. Where most of the "New Women" of Germany had to go to great lengths and great pains to obtain things like proper birth control and abortions, and a few of the more radical had formed their Syndicalist Women's Union in 1920 protesting the "forced labour" of childbearing in reaction— Katharina (a proud and active member since '21) laughed in playful whispers that she'd been "drafted" into the SFB almost a decade before its inception. "Grandmothered in," she chuckled in a coy, breathy whisper that was making Theodor hotter and hotter as she giggled, "so you might say, *daar*-ling . . ."

Theodor showed her a little of what he could do, there in the shadows, going down on her with alacrity and ardour as she gasped and giggled, her tasselled, silky skirt draped over his undulating head; but soon, she wanted him inside her, something she whispered in her hot and eager voice, pulling her skirt to her navel and his head by its hair up to face her, her hands ripping the zip of his rough denim trousers open and welcoming his already hard, pulsing, hungry manhood into the delicious warm folds of her long-sopping sex—her skirt and his trousers left on, loosened just enough, in case they had to make a quick escape. But the Gods and Goddesses of Sex were merciful that night, Eros in all Her hundred forms: the young, rebel couple were unmolested by Bullen or passers-by. Theodor came into a readiness that lasted a good long while, pleasing both himself and his lover till both of them came, almost at once. Katharina's sounds were hot and hungry, a gradual groaning of almost pain in her frustration to come, rewarding and inspiring Theodor to thrust deeper and deeper, dancing and gyrating till her every inner fold felt his touch. Then, all at once, a great shout of ecstatic joy rang throughout the park, echoing in their heads and hearts minutes and minutes later. Theodor cried, too, a great high yelp of pleasure in her deep roar, and lay within her for many moments till he'd grown completely soft again, relishing the hot wet rapture of connection which needn't end with their orgasms. Finally he pulled out and lay beside her on the bench, breathing hard.

Katharina smiled to him, taking his head to her breast, whispering that he'd been a good and faithful lover, one that need fear no inadequacy. She would never have known it was his first time.

Theodor didn't know if he quite believed this; but it was wonderful, overall, so he didn't question it. They lay there till the first light came in a cloudy, early winter grey. Then, it was time to part ways, time to find their separate slumbers in the crazy symphony of a cityscape, miles and miles apart.

They vowed to meet again.

Chapter 4

The next months saw an increasingly dire situation for the economy of Deutschland, and with it many opportunities to build something better. This, at least, was how Theodor saw it, he and his KPD comrades. As the year turned from '22 to '23, the Weimar government of Germany, pressed with runaway inflation and widespread resentment of the vicious reparations payments demanded by the victors of the Great War, ruled to abandon its payments to the banks of France and England. That was in the first half of January. By the middle of January, just days later, French and Belgian troops had occupied the Ruhr valley, threatening renewed invasion of the German heartland. Cuno's and Ebert's government of centrists and bogus socialists effetely urged "passive resistance" against the invasion. In answer, the people rose in strikes, demonstrations, even near riots over the next weeks. People from all classes—but especially the poorer ones—turned out to demand an end to these humiliating (and bankrupting) payments of the vicious tribute. Many clamoured for war again. But many others sounded the clarion unheard since the Bavarian rising of '19, of violent and international revolution as the only solution for the common people on both sides of the Ruhr and the Rhine. *Death to Bankers—French **and** German!* became a familiar cry, and a familiarly reasoned argument in the beer halls and the coffee shops, in the cheap cafeterias and on the bread lines and in the soup kitchens in the cellars of the churches. The KPD newspaper, *Die Rote Fahne,* rode this wave of revolutionary anger, urging workers to "Fight Poincare and Cuno on the Ruhr and on the Spree!"—the headline equating the French government and the German government as alike enemies to the working people of Germany. Meanwhile, there were more and more desperate former peasants from Bavaria and other parts of the countryside, shacking up in makeshift shanties in the public parks and in the back alleys of Berlin. You could see dozens of young men on nearly every street corner now, sitting or lying in gutters amidst the waifs clinging to their mothers in their rags, sharing butts of ragged cigarettes among them, digging in dustbins for scraps of sandwiches or sausages or the unfinished dregs of castaway bottles of beer.

And, as much as there were Spartakists, and Socialists, and anarchists and syndicalists spreading their propaganda and offering their solutions to the crisis, too there were government agents, spies,

Bullen uniformed and Bullen plain-clothes and Bullen undercover, conspiring to thwart the rebellions, blackmailing and informing and inciting false putsches as agents-provocateurs, killing the Revolution stillborn in the womb.

And, too, there were the fascists.

Katharina and Theodor went to separate meetings before meeting one another in late-night cafés and rathskeller bars to continue their flowering relationship, understanding and accepting they were of markedly different politics, however much they felt they were comrades. Their tryst in the park at the beginning of the winter birthed many more as the weather grew colder, then warmed again. The spring came early in '23, days of springtime as early as February, and by the beginning of March the spring weather seemed there for good. In the beginning weeks of their relationship, Katharina and Theodor's love life was very much the same as any young girl and boy throughout the ages. But as their relationship deepened and aged, as some fine cognac Katharina would trade sexual favours for to a corrupt official in the Custom's Office (a cast-off client of Johanna), their sexuality broadened to include all the dark, joyful perversities Katharina had long embraced, but which for Theodor were new. He found that she'd long been what was called a "demi-castor," a daughter of the wealthy classes who supplemented her family stipend by working the sex trade. At first she'd worked in the high class prostitution establishments of the West End, her first years away from home, right after the war. Later, after a brief, half-hearted stint in a sleazier whorehouse in the Alex, she'd found the courage to work the streets, picking up tourists in the Wittenberg Platz who'd come to Berlin to taste the forbidden fruit of Weimar beauty in the ruins. Then, with her new friend Johanna beside her, she'd crossed the blocks to the corner of Passauer and Anbacher streets, in matching poisonous-green boots, symbolizing the dark fetish of psychological enslavement, as well as the many other boot-colour and lace-colour codes for spanking, whipping, collaring, forced feminization, verbal humiliation, smothering in stocking feet—brick red, blood red, gold, brown, cobalt blue, laced in gold, white, black, maroon—all the dark rainbow of colours she and Johanna had lined up in their shared digs. Though Katharina sometimes worked as a domina with her longtime lover, her real preference was toward the masochist, and she'd use the johns that came to her to get off on being helpless and abused by them before duty called to flip them (the meaning of the white ribbons on her boots). Her favourite thing was to work the corners beside Johanna, and be offered by her as a slave the johns could abuse whilst they themselves knelt before Johanna's unforgiving signal whip.

At first, Theodor felt squeamish issuing orders, spanking or slapping Katharina as she craved. But over time, he learned the lesson she wished to teach him, that his masculinity was not a liability, not something to rein in as his Church-ridden and Freud-ridden culture had taught him all his life, but was something which he could unleash and explore without fear or shame. She taught him to top her, led him gently by the hand to a place where she could submit to him utterly, and where he could let himself explore fantasies which he'd not even acknowledged in himself before. For the time that he was slowly discovering his domino side, Katharina continued to offer herself to men and women as a "racehorse," a masochist-slut working at one of the "Institutes for Foreign Language Instruction"—covert brothels of a very specialized type, whose "classrooms" featured bondage equipment hidden behind walls of lockers in the back. She only moderately needed the fees the "students" paid to slap her, to spank her, to bind her and beat her on the spanking benches and the St. Andrew's crosses. Mostly, it was to serve her own pleasure, and as Theodor became more comfortable and more adept, she frequented them less and less. Still, though, in their early relationship, and as more or less a constant, the couple embraced an open-ended form, which allowed for multiple lovers while retaining a very real commitment to one another.

For some reason, though, Theo's love life with men was slow in the making. This was somewhat from lack of opportunity (male homosexuality was still illegal under Article 175 of the Weimar Legal Code, whilst lesbianism was not, making the gay-boy bars and clubs more dangerous from police raids and making "out" men more a rarity than out women), and somewhat from Theo's uncertainty as to what he really wanted.

"There's no pressure, liebling," Katharina assured. "While I'd love to see some young fairy-stud ream you from behind, or some old daddy suck you till you scream his name and beg to return the gesture—I think we've time to be choosy. I only want someone my suße *really* wants to break that fag cherry of his with. . . ."

Knowing how beautiful it was to break his straight cherry, and how long—nineteen long years—it took to find the right person to break it with, Theodor felt no great hurry. Everything would come, in its time . . .

For the time being, however, they lived and loved in the shadows—the shadows of their homophobic government, the shadows of the laws against prostitution and drugs and most forms of joy as they saw it, the shadows of the differing and divergent political movements from monarchism to fascism to communism to anarchism to the grim static normalcy of the liberal-socialist status quo. Katharina took no man's word as her own, her small cell meetings of shifting groups, forming now, now dissolving, now forming again—always a group of individualists, following their own visions, however "collectivist" the little groups often were in name and theory.   Theodor for his part took the sage advice of Old Max, given fatherly to him before the Communist cell meetings which of course his lover did not attend, advice about this and that, politics and friendship and love (this last edited for "proletarian consumption," Theo chuckled to himself). Old Max gave advice to all the young men and women of the cell, and it was taken as fatherly counsel by most all of them. Yet, thinking on it, Theodor and his young comrades were coming to notice how, in the meetings proper, most of what Max and the other Old Guard Spartakists related to the Youth Brigade was not advice, but rather straightforward directives—*orders*—and these seemed far less wise. Max had a way of grinning a kind of groaning grin, a sigh of sympathy for the young men and women to whom he was relaying the communiqués he got from the Zentrale (the Central Committee) of the Deutschland-wide KPD; he'd shrug his shoulders and turn his smiling head a little to the side, and say, "What else can we do, comrades? *C'est la guerre, nicht wahr*?" These orders coming from on high were in turn coming from Moscow—and who but fascists, bourgeois, and stupid, silly anarchists would dare question Moscow now? If we wanted to spread the Workers' Revolution here to Deutschland, and from here to all Europe—well, then, it wouldn't do to question now, to break ranks, would it? At this point in history, Max intoned, to break the chain of command was tantamount to working for the other side.

But Old Max knew, and he said it with that smile, that the orders coming down from the Zentrale were sometimes hard to follow. The party line was very difficult to tow, especially as the events of the year were growing more and more tumultuous and confusing. As the year surged forward from the early, blustery spring to a broiling summer, the value of the Mark plummeted. Inflation was such that, by September, people were literally carrying their paper money in wheelbarrows to the shops to buy a few groceries. It became common for workplaces round the city to let the workers have an extended mid-morning lunch—not to *eat*, but to rush to the shops to buy the necessaries that by day's end their wages would no longer purchase. Grocers went through their stores twice or thrice or more times each day, pulling off price tags, sticking new ones on—and those numbers were each time higher than the day—or even the *hour*—before. It became such a ponderous task to keep up with the changing prices that whole shifts of people were hired just to walk round the stores, putting zeroes at the ends of price-tags. A loaf of bread that cost a few marks a year ago climbed to tens and then hundreds, till by this perilous September, it had climbed to literally over a million. That number would go up into the *trillions* by November—all for the same loaf of bread. People with possessions—petty-bourgeois with pianos, silver tea services, jewellery—*anything*—were trading them to peasants and farmers in the countryside just for basic meat, milk, eggs, cheese. And most everyone else became vegetarians, all over Germany, regardless of their ethics or politics.

Throughout this tumultuous, insane period, the KPD comrades were ordered not to pilfer. Stealing was anarchy, it was reasoned from on high. And though everyone did it—Theodor included—from time to time just to survive, they did it in whispers. The guilt of "sinning" thus was worse for the Communists than for those who were merely Catholic or Protestant. Sin was all around, and no one could escape it, none help but fall into its snare. Yet, it couldn't be discussed openly. The hypocrisy, and the paranoia, became part of the "cross" Theodor and his friends had to bear.

The worst thing of all, though, was the line coming down from the upper circles that the Social Democrats were now to be considered the new, real enemy of the Communists. Moscow was urging all the good comrades to call them "Social-Fascists" in their everyday discourse with the political and non-political alike, and in fact to see them as more of a threat even than the avowed fascists, the growing Nazi Party. The Brownshirts were everywhere lately, picking fights on the streets, harassing passers-by, and—*increasingly*—fucking with KPD meetings. The worst of the many "orders" that were coming down from the Zentrale, the hardest of all to follow, was a general refusal to attack and break up the fascists' meetings in retaliation for what was going on in the KPD cells all over town.

It really was ridiculous. And a lot of Theodor's young brothers were throwing rocks through Nazi windows, slashing tires of known Brownshirt cars, and generally giving what-for to the thugs—whenever and wherever it was called for. But like so much else, they acted in these ways against the orders of their superiors. "Tolerance" or "pacifism" were certainly not the lines being expressly handed down by the Party. Indeed, workers' militias, called "the hundreds," had been forming for a while now, their stated purpose to defend working people against fascist and government reprisals during the strikes that erupted all over Germany by the mid-year and forced Cuno from power. If Comrade Lenin (who, they said, was feeling sickly of late—though this was just rumour, and likewise could not be openly talked about) had actually urged anything like pacifism, it would have been no time at all before his enraged followers in Germany crossed over to the ranks of the ultra-left Communist Workers' Party, or perhaps even to the anarchists. But the line being presented, and fought for by the higher-ups, becoming mandatory amongst all circles below them, was that it was the SPD that was really the problem. Therefore, it was in the factories, on the shop floors, at the demonstrations, in the unions, and through the elections, that the fighting should be done. Everyone would certainly see the foolish idiocy of the Nazi propaganda for what it was, it was said from on high. Much more dangerous, they said, were the other, rival Socialists, who could actually claim real working class politics in their theoretical arsenal, had a long working class history, and still had a large working class base of support. Fight *them*, cut *their* head off the proletarian mass, and the Communists would be the obvious choice of the working class in Germany.

Again and again, it was drilled into Theodor, this need to win the battle between the rival socialisms. National Socialism so obviously *wasn't* a socialism, that the Nazis (it was advised, ever so sagely) would soon dig their own graves, and bury themselves beneath the garbage heap of history. The "United Front" against the Fascists that so many people were proposing, the one that was hoped for in that demonstration where Theodor had met Katharina the year before, was not to be countenanced by Comrade Lenin, Comrade Trotsky, Comrades Radek and Zinoviev and Bukharin. Thus, not to be countenanced by the German Communists' Central

Committee, who, though once independent of Moscow and still claiming to be, fell more and more in line with the Russian comrades, an increasing conformity throughout the Third International. And therefore, the order went, not to be even idly talked about by any of the rank-and-file comrades, like Theodor, unless and until the Party agreed to change the policy in the open debates at their Congress scheduled for the anniversary of the October Revolution in Moscow.

"You'll have a voice, then, comrade," Old Max smiled to him, and to each frustrated, angry young man and woman he had to convince over those months. "Until then—if you really take issue with the Party line, and have a substantiated, genuine minority view—then, *argue for it!* Argue for it, within the ranks of the Party! That's how things change, comrade. That's the 'democratic' part of Democratic Centralism, eh? I mean, write a position paper, and present it to the Congress this fall . . ."

Theodor Priser decided to take the task upon himself. He started writing just such a position paper, arguing for a mobilization of the hundreds to take the offensive against the fascists and entice SPD-affiliated workers to join them, writing it with two of his friends, a freckled, flame-haired, gregarious and articulate if uneducated fellow who worked with him at the warehouse named Klaus, and a quiet, dark, and studious older Polish girl named Nadia. It was the first pamphlet he'd ever compose. But he'd not present it to anyone till well after the Party Congress, because the notes he and his two friends began making together at the end of those meetings did not survive the fire-bombing in September.

Maximilian and the other old guys were gone, the meeting over, their business done. Theodor, Klaus, Nadia, and a dozen others of the Youth Brigade had all lingered in the office that afternoon, talking of the recent strikes, the possibilities of risings in Hamburg and Munich and down in Bavaria, sharing round a cigarette rolled from shredded bits of an old cabbage leaf found in a dustbin, scribbling notes on the backs of the new, high-denomination marks whose blank backs were cheaper to waste than notepaper, sketching lazy doodles there, when a flurry of rocks came flying through the windows. Bottles of petrol with burning rags stuffed in their necks followed by the score, setting the whole office ablaze in a few tens of seconds. When the comrades pushed their way through the glass onto the street, they found nearly twice their number in the stupid, deceptively frumpy uniforms of the SA waiting for them.

The battle was short. Klaus and five or six others each wrested bits of glass from the windows they'd crawled through, their hands bound in work-gloves or the tatters of their shirts—makeshift knives against the fascists. But the fascists had clubs and sticks, and before the drone of the polizei sirens came sounding from the boulevard, the store front office was burnt-out wreckage, and seven of the comrades were on the pavement, unconscious, with broken ribs or broken heads, bleeding into the gutter. Theodor and Klaus and a few others had managed to stay on their feet till the polizei arrived, all the Brownshirts who they hadn't flattened fleeing the scene just before the Bullen came, as if they somehow knew when the cops would arrive. Nadia, who had braved the flames and gone back into the office to save the records and the monies of their cell, emerged coughing and grimy with ashes, her black hair wild and singed, her long dress scorched and tattered. She looked to her fellow pamphleteers as a doctor to the mother of a stillborn baby, ashy, inky shreds of what had been months of work sticking from a mangled double-drum rotary cyclostyle—the only print-copier the comrades had. Rather than listen to their explanations—rather, certainly, than listen to their urgings to do something about the damaged property or the damaged young people—the Bullen arrested the lot of them, shoving them in their uncannily numerous paddy-wagons and holding them hours into the night.

The rendezvous Theodor was to keep with his lover in a café in the Mitte, near where the rivers converged with the canal, midway between their respective organizing meetings, was not kept that night. And Katharina knew to look first to the hospitals, then to the jail, to find her lover. She somehow secured his bail, and the other comrades of the Youth Brigade who'd been arrested, winning them to a measure of the anarchist cause without ever making an argument. Old Max didn't arrive at the jail till the next morning, claiming not to have heard about it all.

"You're fraulein's a good one, there, Theodor," enthused Klaus, and Nadia agreed. They wanted to have a drink before they went home that night, and Katharina offered to buy them a round at her favourite watering hole, a nondescript rathskeller a good walk south and east from the bustling Potsdamer Platz, a place very easily missed amidst the dives of the Jagerstraße, called The Black Tie. None of Theodor's friends had ever been there, and they soon realized why: it was a tavern crawling with drunken anarchists, of all the various circles in the city, a place where the KPD and the SPD looked very much alike to the patrons. Though anarchist circles were small in Berlin, it seemed they all came here of a midnight, to drink the health of Makhno, who had escaped the commies in the Ukraine and was safely exiled in Paris. Makhno, the first fellow to wear the black tie—though never, *never* round his neck.

The Black Tie was ironically named, especially if you didn't know the history of the colour politically, that black was the hue of the anarchist banner (not the now-co-opted red), that Mahkno's peasant army in the Ukraine had till just three years ago defended the last of the Revolution from both the czarist White Army and the Red Army of the murderer Trotsky, under a black banner. Most of the people who drank here, if not anarchists, were vagabonds and drifters, disreputable types in almost any company, whose shirts often did not even have proper collars, let alone ties. The Communists who'd come to drink on the nice lady who'd bought their freedom mostly drank quickly and exited, not liking the dirty cellar, the people drinking there, or the implications. Nadia excused herself, binding her black hair back into the tight bun she'd lost over the long evening, promising rather formally to pay the stranger Katharina back her bail money—a promise she kept within a fortnight. Klaus alone stuck around, for he was a lady's man even more surely than a party comrade, and there were a trio of pretty Chontes in a corner, Polish-Jewish prostitutes hailing from Lublin, just getting off work that night, whom he found pleasant company, impressing them with his recent tales of fighting and jail—all for the right reasons. Without the eye of any but the most forgiving of his comrades, Theodor finally relaxed, and drank of Katharina's lips like a bottle of prized wine.

"You okay, suβe?" she asked him, kissing his blackened eye over and over and seeing that he had a good showering of lager to kill the pain.

"Yeah, I think so. . . . How was your meeting?"

"Better than yours, I know."

"Yeah, well. Actually, the meeting itself wasn't bad today. Over the last weeks, we've been studying the Labour Theory of Value and how it applies to the current economic crisis. It's been a good discussion, actually."

"Yes, love."

"What've you people been talking about?"

"Oh, the exact same bullshit."

"You've been talking about Marxist economics?"

His smile was too quizzical for condescension. They'd already been through all the debates of the value of "theory" and "dialectics" and the like, and had long agreed to differ. Her boldness was not uncharacteristic; but after tonight, everything seemed much more important, and much less, than it had ever been.

"Well, liebling," she sighed and stretched, "we anarchists have our own little inside jokes, too. You debate the dialectical this versus the synthetical that; we talk about individual this versus the collective that. I actually got quite sick of it all, after a while. If it weren't for the beer and the mulligan stew, I think I'd drop out of meetings altogether."

"You—*drink*, at meetings?"

"And eat. How else would they get us to come back to 'em? Why? Don't you guys lubricate your mental gears with a little *aqua vitae*, during your oh-so-pressing economic discussions?"

"Well . . . no. There's a sobriety rule at our meetings. The idea is that, to raise your consciousness, it helps to be conscious. Not a bad thing, really . . ."

She laughed at him suddenly.

"What?"

"Oh, my fucking Lord, Theo! No wonder you people don't grow at all! You know what the fucking Nazis have on all you guys? They give people what they want. Their meetings are like Oktoberfest every night! They get 'em good and drunk, and then they talk their garbage, and by then nobody bothers to argue with it."

"Well, that's why the Nazis are gonna fail. Their politics are just thuggishness. Drunken, stupid, backward thuggishness. We've got the politics that can really emancipate this working class, Katharina. What the hell do they got?"

"Fun! That's the sad truth of it, Theo, love! Most people don't want to come to meetings when they could go to the flicks, or the cabarets, or the beer halls. I was just telling my 'serious' comrades about that tonight. You know, we've got that debate goin' on, too, about 'organizational unity,' and 'seriousness,' and all that Nechaev-ish 'giving up everything for the Revolution' nonsense, too. The Nazis—damn them to blazes!—they understand that most people don't go for all that cold, intellectual bullshit. They *work* all day, brother! They don't want to go to some boring lecture about economics with their few good hours of the week. And they don't want that formal, 'committee' structure invading all their free-time either. They want to enjoy themselves! Mind you, I don't mind planning an action, or spreading a message. But, when ya come down to it, Theo—if there's not a—a *human* element in it—a warm, sensuous, funny, *real* element in it—then politics—of *any* kind!—is doomed to repeat all the ugliness of the last centuries of this civilised delusion. It's not my kinda politics. And it's nobody's kinda politics, if they've got an ounce of self-respect or self-love in their souls!"

Theodor realized Katharina was drunker than he was—and he'd had a good half-dozen lagers by this point. He could not tell if she were angry with him, or with some other person or thing—but it was clear she was angry. Gently, he told her his objection to what she was saying, imagining he was siding with whatever or whomever she'd argued with, probably at her meeting this very night. But his night had been rough, and he was only a human being, too. Dialectics, and theory, and the party line, were not things he wished to take lightly right now. He'd very nearly gotten his head kicked in earlier for his allegiance to them.

"If you're not serious, Katharina, who will you convince? You anarchists might have more 'fun' at your meetings, but what—*practically*—do any of you do? I mean, the people who adhere to your philosophy in this town probably aren't enough to fill this bar at a peak hour! We Communists might not be filling the streets right now—but the *workers* are—and *will!* Mark me, sister—give 'em a month, or maybe two on the outside—and we'll have a real revolutionary crisis in this country. And when people rise—they fight! And they die!! That's *serious shit*, fraulein! It's not time to be drunk, and disorganized, and—"

"—My *God*, Theo! People go out in the streets for as many reasons as there are people out there! They go out because of *passion—anger*, maybe even *hate*—all mixed up with *hope, vision—LOVE!!* They're not gonna go out there because of some interesting little thing they read about in a book, comrade! They're not gonna leave your boring old lecture hall saying—'Jesu Maria! That algebraic equation I studied tonight about use-value and exchange-value really motivates me to go sock those Bullen in the eye!' God!! You sound like those fucking platform people at the meeting tonight!"

"Well, I don't really know what that means, but I'm sorry I

sound like someone you're not happy with. Seems to me, though, that theory is *exactly* what people value. What inspires them. Hell! It inspires me!"

"Okay, Theo, okay. But that's *your* turn-on. And, you know, let the platform people, and the commies, and all y'all masturbate with your braincells all ya want. Get together and circle-jerk each other to atheist heaven! It doesn't matter who's wrong or right. It just matters what people actually *do.*"

"So what do we do?!"

She smiled, wisely, daringly.

"What do you *want* to do, Theo? What does that fellow talking to those girls who came with you want to do right now? What *should* you all be doing, after this horrid afternoon?

"Well, I'll tell you what *we're* gonna do: we're gonna all get good and stiff here at the Black Tie, so we feel *no pain.* And then, we're gonna go bust up one of the goddamn *Nazi meetings.* What d'ya say?"

Theodor instantly saw the "seriousness" of his "flighty" comrade now. He sensed then that his intoxicated, illogical state might just be the best one for doing the serious work his Party, with all its reasoned platform, forbade him to do. He looked to Klaus, that simple fellow talking to those girls about anything but serious politics, kissing one, then the other, then the other, giggling light-hearted and free, and knew he could convince him of this most important duty which he was prepared to defy his elder comrades to perform. He was just drunk enough, just angry enough, to be open to the course of action he would tomorrow probably regret. He was just fucked up enough to do the one thing in the world that was not fucked up.

"Who's all in this, sister?" he said softly.

She grinned.

"Hell, Theo, darling! I'm ready to go, just you and me! But, I bet I could get half this bar to go with us. And I don't give a rat's ass how many people 'agree' with my little cell's 'points of unity.' Let's get all the bums and the sailors and the fags and the whores together—and let's beat the fuck out of those lousy bastards for once!—even if we get killed tryin'!!"

He looked at her.

"Fuck yeah, sister," he breathed. "Fuck yeah."

She kissed him deeply, stirring something primal in him; then she wobbled off to her circle of friends round a table in the back. He got up and stumbled over to Klaus.

"Hey comrade," he smiled. "What say we get back at those Nazi pigs tonight?"

Klaus looked cloudily to him from where he leaned on the prettiest woman's shoulder. It was as if he'd been having the same discussion with them for the past quarter hour.

"Man," he said low, "we might be kicked outta the Party."

"So what?"

Klaus thought a second or two, but no longer. He drank down the rest of his beer in a gulp, kissed each woman at his side, and bade them all *adieu*. The one he kissed last, prettier, braver than her companions, a titian-haired, zaftig beauty with some hard muscle in her soft, curvy flesh, rose to join him. They came to Theodor's side.

Somebody with a squeezebox started playing a familiar strain, a fight song strikers sang back in the last century, before the International split between anarchist, socialist, and communist, when they all marched together. A song Theodor's Papa must have sung when the old man was younger than Theo was now, when the SPD still meant something.

There was no rallying speech, no calls for united action; but in a few minutes, some twenty people, mostly tramps and vagabonds looking for a little angry fun, had joined Katharina and Theo and Klaus and Klaus' new friend on the street outside the rathskeller. Theo couldn't tell the "serious revolutionaries" from the hooligans, who among the score of angry men and women were anarchists proper and who were just riled up drunks—but he realized theoretical unity was not a prerequisite for action. Without a word—or rather, with many, laughing and cursing, the score marched down an alley to the place where one of the whores said her pimp would be tonight (pimps, like soured, bankrupt businessmen and unemployed university professors, made up the bulk of the Brownshirts' rank and file, Theo would later learn). Rounding a corner, the twenty slowed down, most of them having armed themselves with chair-legs and chains and broken, jagged bottles found in the dustbins, or bits of branches ripped off dead, rotten trees. They grouped themselves together outside the little hall, hearing the Nazis singing a drunken strain of what had been an old leftist fight song of the 1848 German Revolutions, *"Das Heckerlied,"*—rewritten by the Nazis to reflect their lousy propaganda.

Sharpen the long knives on the pavement, the strain echoed down the alley, *let the knives stab into the Jews' body! Blood must flow extreme extensive! And we shit on the freedom of this Jews' Republic!*

An old, half-blind bum, a grizzled, bearded veteran not of the last War, but of the now forgotten Franco-Prussian War of more than a generation past, stumbled half-lame to the front of the place, and hurled a brick through the front window. He stood there, taunting and cursing as the Nazis within rushed toward the front of their hall. That's when everyone else busted down the side door and flooded in from the back.

The Brownshirts still looked out to the front where the brick had fallen, and while their backs were all turned, the anarchists, whores, and tramps rushed them from behind. One of them, Theo recognized, was the ugly, big thug Gretchen had dumped him for, and he took great pleasure in knocking him to the floor with the rusty crowbar somebody handed him.

There were considerably more than twenty people at the Nazi meeting, maybe as many as thrice more. But the tramps and the whores and the anarchists had caught them off guard. Many of the Nazis' people were slumped over long tables, near-drowned in cheap beer, and before they could get up to fight, the tables and the beer had all been overturned, and most of the fools found themselves knocked to the floor amidst the frothy flood and broken glass.

Katharina was a flurry of kicks, fists, and vicious biting. Theodor thought to defend her, but she needed no help. Blood was flying everywhere, the swastika flags kicked over and trampled, the many pamphlets informing of the "Protocols of the Elders of Zion" and all their other rubbish scattered like confetti at a ticker-tape parade. Theodor, who had been a fighter as much as a proletarian male had to be growing up, but no more than that, found an unexpected thrill at clobbering so many bastards, and he thrilled no less than he would have had this been the first battle of the Great Revolution.   In a way, it was . . .

The whole thing was over in five minutes, maybe less. By the time the tramps regrouped outside, then fled the sirens of the polizei, most of the Brownshirts and their stupid followers were knocked out amidst the shattered beer steins and ruined pamphlets. Some of the tramps had gotten their share of blows, too, and smarted sorely the next morning. But Nazis, like all bullies, were cowards, and a lot of the able-bodied Brownshirts had fled into the night, fearing the fair, unfair fight they were losing, and the Bullen who came to sort out the wreckage.

The next morning found Theo passed out in Katharina's arms, half lying and half dangling off the oriental divan, and Klaus making drunken love to the prettiest of last night's Chontes on the floor, their shared auburn hair falling, sweaty and tickly into their shared black eyes, and the burning of their India-ink sailor's tattoos of each other's names they'd gotten on their asses in the blurry blackout haze after their victory making them giggle, along with the fun, painful pleasures of hard, drunken fucking. Ten or fifteen new friends were lying among them, sleeping satisfied, if sore sleeps, till well into the afternoon. There was a meeting to go to, a Communist meeting in another hall across the city. But both loyal comrades found good excuses for missing it.

Chapter 5

Katharina lay back on the armless sofa, meditating on the indentations on the plaster ceiling of her analyst's office. Sunlight, a drearily bright overcast autumnal white, paling everything to a colourless montage, bathed the office, the desk, the placards of psychiatric achievement, the bookcase, the plant, the skeleton clock, Katharina, and the man whose manner and countenance suggested uncannily the portrait of Freud hanging beside a seascape on the wall. Everything was panelling, shag carpet, and silence. The only sound was the ticking of that clock, as the doctor sat there, waiting for Katharina to start.

"I've had that dream again," she said, perfunctorily, because she did not know what else to say.

"Which dream?" husked the refined, Austrian accent beside her.

"The one about travelling."

"The one about the train?"

"That's right."

"What did it signify this time, do you think?"

Katharina had been plagued by dreams, mostly the same one, recurring and recurring, of trying to get to the train station, and failing to get there, or being on a train, and realizing too late she was going in the wrong direction. Always, always it was the same. Katharina thought at times the man she saw was a fraud. Freudian theories were of only dubious efficacy in her mind, and he was a textbook case of an analyst who used textbooks too much. Shouldn't *he* be trying to figure out her dream's significance? Why was *she* always asked to do it? Why, in short, was she paying him?

"One different thing, this time," she sighed, "is that Theo was on the train with me."

"Theo, the young man you've been seeing over this last year?"

"That's right."

"What was this young man doing, in the dream?"

"He was . . . sitting with me. That's all. It was . . . comforting."

"Why, comforting?"

"Because, I . . . wasn't alone."

The old man scribbled something down on a pad in his lap. Then, there was that profound and awkward silence. Katharina was supposed to elaborate, to direct the conversation she herself was having. Just today, though, she'd tired of the charade. She just sat there, saying nothing. Fully five minutes went by. At last, she broke out laughing.

"Why are you laughing, Katharina?"

"Because, doctor, you're funny!"

"Why do you find me funny?"

"Because you never have anything to say!"

"Katharina, this therapy is designed to elicit responses from you. It would be . . . heavy-handed . . . to direct things too closely."

"Perhaps. But, you don't direct things at all."

"That is my preferred method."

"Why?"

"This is not the place to ask me questions, Katharina. Questions are meant for *your* treatment."

Katharina sighed in frustration. This was the sixth analyst she'd seen in not twice that many months, and there'd been others before. From just before she'd met Theo late in the last autumn to this October, she'd been an almost daily communicant of the rites of Freud and his apostles. As a child, she'd been referred to such doctors by her mother, who believed her sick in body and mind, as well as, if the mother or she had been believers in such metaphysics, her soul. Her brothers, one younger and one older, would have to carry on the family name. Katharina herself was a lost cause, at least according to her family, sterilized by suggestion of those same childhood doctors, and more than once committed for extended stays on psychiatric wards—until her great aunt had spirited her away and taken the young teenager with her on a world tour, from the Swiss Alps to the Riviera to Morocco and on to North and Latin America.

Lately, Katharina had found her own solace in it. Having been long condemned to seeing these doctors, these analysts, she used them now voluntarily, as an opportunity for her own growth—in spite of whatever agendas they might be advancing. It seemed right, fitting that she'd had these torrid dalliances with the apostles of Freud. She thought to a favourite heroine she'd been reading of in just the last few months, Metta Rudloff, that Weirauch character she felt so many parallels with, how early on she was crazy—strangling her adult caretaker when she was just a little girl, just as Katharina had many times longed to do. Tortured between extremes, just like Katharina, Metta was: wanting to be as the loving

Christ one day, then despising all humanity the next, wondering whether she should be a sexless nun or the ravisher who could seduce the whole world—wanting to leave corporeality and become part of the ether, to become a superhuman being—or whether it would not, after all, be pleasanter to be dead and gone. *The Scorpion* trilogy were the novels of lust and longing which spoke most to Katharina's heart of late—most certainly to her moods, which defied normality and dared for maddened transcendence in this earthly life. The longing for souls no longer in this world, impossible loves she found herself fantasizing and dreaming about, people like Dolorosa, pen-name of the mysterious Maria Eichhorn, who had lived as both a dominatrix and a submissive in the years round the turn of the century—had written liltingly pornographic cabaret poetry and been a chanteuse of cabaret songs to celebrate it all—only to lose herself somewhere in Istanbul in 1907 or 1908, never to be heard from again . . . This was what the Scorpion Olga Rado had told Katharina's heroine Metta really turned her on—a necrophilia for souls no longer here—a sense that your true love, your soul-mate, might not even live in the same century as you, let alone the same part of the world. Katharina fell into melancholia considering Dolorosa, and Anna Elisabet Weirauch, and the characters that both women had made who never existed. She found herself deeply mourning the loss of those whom she had never, *could* never, have met. Katharina was, in a word, mad. And she saw these psychiatrists and analysts as part of the mad life fate had given her to lead.

But, she'd had bad luck. Almost never had she found an analyst that really clicked with her. Only one time, a young man whose counselling of her ended with his untimely death—a suicide, apparently—had any apostle of the rites of psychiatry truly proved a good fit. That was years ago, now, when she'd just turned thirteen. Most everyone since had been ridiculously inadequate for what she needed. This latest man was but another of the same.

Still, Katharina endeavoured to make it work.

"I like this boy," she said simply.

"What do you like about him?"

"He's . . . different."

"Different from whom? From the other boys you've seen?"

"Yes. Exactly that. He's . . . from the wrong side of the canal."

"Do you mean that he's poor?"

"*Very* poor."

"And you find this rewarding in some way?"

"Yes, I do."

"What do you find rewarding?"

"He's so . . . *pretty.*"

"Do you find him feminine?"

"Yes. And, no."

The doctor did something unexpected, then. He chuckled a little.

"It *is* unusual," he commented, "to find such a—*delicacy,* among the lower classes."

Something about his snicker was distasteful to Katharina. "I don't know about *that,*" she said, in almost protest.

"Well, Katharina, you don't really know the lower classes, do you?"

This was getting all of a sudden quite directive.

"I haven't had much experience with that, no. Not till the last few years. . . . But, it seems to me many people can be pretty."

"Do you find him as a woman, in your attraction?"

The doctor knew of Katharina's dalliances among her own gender; it was one of the first things she'd told him about herself. The psychiatrist judged it all coldly, scientifically, in keeping with the textbooks of the day. He did not know Magnus Hirschfeld or Iwan Bloch, had never heard of Albert Eulenburg, nor certainly Karl Heinrich Ulrichs or Edward Carpenter. He was content with the predominant, prevailing theories on the psyche, on sexuality, and all the many aspects of life that derived from these things. In Katharina's mind, Freud had once been revolutionary; but, times had changed, and while most people were still getting used to his way of looking at things, Katharina herself felt the torch had definitely been passed. Freud was, in her opinion, anti-woman, anti-child, and this to her outweighed his other anti-patriarchal, anti-conservative aspects. Sex was out of the closet, at least a little, thanks in part to him; but, now that it was out of the closet—what was there to do with it? Hirschfeld knew; Carpenter and Weirauch and Dolorosa and a dozen other thinkers, writers, lovers, knew; Katharina knew, too.

The analyst was encouraging, in his impersonal way, of Katharina's dating men, even one as apparently unsavoury as this working class boy. He felt it was her overcoming some complex or other, to function heterosexually. But, Katharina was proud of her complexes, and she knew that her new lover had some of the same complexes. She espied the textbooks lying beside Freud's endless studies on this analyst fellow's bookshelf, as she'd glanced at them endlessly over the weeks of boredom in his office on his couch. The complete works of Carl Westphal sat beside an updated volume of *Psychopathia Sexualis* by Richard von Krafft-Ebing, and she mused on the contrast—two old bastards from the nineteenth century, both of whom would conclude she and Theo and everyone she knew and loved were "sick." Because she was sick, she and her boy, Westphal would have argued that the law had no business with them, that the old Prussian Article 143 (reiterated now by Article 175 of Weimar's Constitution) should not chuck her boy into prison for wanting men. A nice sentiment, that we poor perverts should not be imprisoned; but perverts we remain, Katharina mused, according to those cold, dead scientists.

She laughed at Krafft-Ebing's condemnation of her kind, he who had very much approved of the sodomy laws. He'd theorized all her "hyperesthesia" and "paraesthesia" (the old bugger's words for "too much" sexual desire and the desire for the "wrong" object—*women*, in her case) were due to masturbation at a young age. She laughed again, deflecting the analyst's queries about her laughter, thinking how much she'd delighted in self-love as a girl, how she wouldn't dream of stopping as long as her old withered hands still worked. Krafft-Ebing's nastiness and all the pretty articles in *Die Freundschaft* about Eros came together when she frigged herself, she thought, smiling. The "base" desires and the highest spiritualities met at her centre, her root chakra, as the Hindus would say. There was no contradiction between lust and love, then. All was revelation . . . revolution . . .

"How is your melancholia, lately?" the doctor by turns inquired, after they'd had a pointless cat-and-mouse about Theo's 'femininity.'

Katharina sighed. She knew, of her many "complexes," this was one she at least partly sympathized with her analyst's attempts to rid her of. She did not like her depression. But, what was it, really? Was it so very strange, actually? Or was it simply the natural response of a rational human being to an unnatural and irrational society?

"It's still there," she admitted. "I've actually been dealing with it a lot lately."

"What has caused this bout, do you think?"

"Doctor—it is *you* who are supposedly the expert on all this. I've no idea what gets me down. It just . . . happens."

The analyst scribbled some more things down on the pad in his lap. Then, he looked up at the clock.

"Well, Katharina," he said, humourlessly, passionlessly, "I believe that's all the time we have for today."

"Well, what about my depression?"

"I believe the answer is what I've always said—what others before me have said. You must cultivate a sense of *proportion.*"

"Fuck you."

Katharina said this later, much later, to herself as she sat in her apartment alone, in the further room, looking out at the unlovely street where she lived, at the oily spot on the wall beside the oily curtains that had once been Johanna's butterfly mirror, her teeth clenching a yellow strip of rubber Johanna had once used as a tourniquet, when Vana Tallinn and Russian champagne failed to deaden her enough. She said it to the phantom analyst in her mind, who was a composite of all the analysts she'd ever had over her twenty-two years. She hated this composite person, quite apart from the feelings, mixed as they were, that she harboured toward the persons who made up this composite. They were always telling her the same thing: *proportion.* If she had "proportion," a clear perspective on what was important and what was not, she would get out of her funk, be free of her melancholia. But, what the hell did this mean? It seemed akin to "dialectics," or any of the other useless theories that abounded in her world. She knew what she wanted. She wanted the warmth of sex, of opium, of anarchy. She did not want "proportion." She had no interest in being a "functional member of society." Society was mad. Society was nothing but a highly efficient and brilliantly successful method of industrial mass murder. Every "advance" European civilisation had made in the last centuries had been turned against itself—by the very same methods by which it had been advanced. The science of curing illnesses had created germ warfare. The technologies of railways and telegraphs, linking the world together, had done nothing less than divide the continents of Africa, Asia, and the Americas into slave-colonies. Newspapers, the cinema, recording and radio had opened whole new ways of people's knowing things; but fewer and fewer hands controlled more and more of it—and so disinformation, ignorance, prejudice, and superstitious slaveries either to the hateful mainstream religions or to the growing occult paranoia of charlatans and demagogues had been spread through the population with dizzying speed and damning power. *This* was society. To "function" in such a society was to be insane—and, despite her many problems, sanity was among the few things Katharina cherished in herself.

Johanna had been gone now over a week. She'd taken her liqueurs and her perfumes, her jewellery and her records, her books and her boots. She'd probably already found herself some other place to live. There'd been no goodbyes. But, wasn't that the way things always were? People came into Katharina's life, and then disappeared, just as quickly, without trace. She had other friends, of course, and looked forward to the night, when they would all come over, and keep her company. But, how many of them could really keep her company? They were hail-fellows-well-met, not bosom comrades, she thought bitterly. Some of them, it was true, seemed to care. But they were all caught up in their scene, the same scene she herself was caught up in. The focus was not to care, but to experience, experience as much of life as you could. Then, there was the work, of propaganda, both of the word and the deed. There were those among her scene who were quite serious about this, and they tended to look askance on the other, more "frivolous" members of their circle. But they were of little comfort, either. Cold comfort, her friends, she thought then, biting the rubber, breathing its scent. It was all such a cold thing, really . . .

"No!" she cursed her thoughts. She hated when she got on this tangent. It made all the things that were beautiful into something ugly, sinister. She thought of art, of literature, of all the things her friends had made that had lifted her out of her morass and had made her love the world again. She thought of the private art collection her family had of great artists past, that her mother was so proud of, that her father had acquired at such expense. It was tasteful; it was aesthetically pleasing; some of it was truly beautiful. But it was horrible. It was so much debris from a class she hated being part of. Cultural debris. Garbage. And what was modern art but newer garbage, desperate, feeble attempts to depict a desperate, enfeebled world—or abandon depiction altogether, as if to give up the duty to try? Dada had faded, fizzling out in just the last year, and whatever would come next was destined just to fade in turn. Endless endlessness, revolts against revolts against revolts—and nothing ever changed anyone's minds for long. It was all just destined for the walls of the "hepper," savvier rich collectors in the coming, pointless generations . . .

"NO!!!"

She found herself weeping.

There was a knock at the door.

Sighing hard, she picked herself up from the rocker where Johanna had sat, extricating her ass from the embroidered, silken cushions and her legs from the plush ottoman that all seemed to grasp at her like some kind of vice, the vice of pleasure, of comfort, of privilege—God! How she hated herself!

She wiped her eyes and opened the door, the door she'd paid extra to have installed there, to keep out the noise of the tenement, to cheat the gods of poverty she pretended to embrace their measure of her inconvenience—to find the one person she did not despise. Theodor stood there.

"Theo!" she smiled, jumping into his arms. "Thank God you're here!"

Theodor laughed, and shook her as she splayed in his arms. He kissed her. Then, he carried her over the threshold. The door was again shut, again locked.

"How are you, good comrade?" he smiled.

She smiled to him.

"Comrade," she repeated. "Yeah, brother. That's what we are—*comrades*—*Comrades to the End!* . . . What brings you over here so early in the afternoon?"

Theodor laughed, looking down.

"I got fired," he said. He didn't seem all that displeased.

"I'm so sorry, Theo!"

"Naw, that's okay. I hated working at that place, anyway. . . . Where's Johanna?"

They were standing in the parlour. Katharina took him by the hand, and led him into the further room. She shut the double doors, though nobody was there to claim privacy from. She told him that she had no idea where the bitch got off to.

"Bitch, huh?" Theodor chuckled, dropping his kitbag on the floor and tossing off his jacket. "Things not so good in the land of domestic bliss, eh?"

"Oh, domestic bliss my ass! She's a domineering fucking fascist! That's what she is. I *hate* her, I think."

Theodor nodded sympathetically, but not entirely with

understanding. She changed the subject, to the last of her cigarettes dipped in opium. She offered to share it with Theodor, and he accepted.

They smoked their cigarette. Then, without a word, they made love. It was beautiful, their lovemaking, such that Katharina was quite brought out of her melancholia for a time. He took the part of her master, her joyful bottoming encouraging every rough, unacknowledged domineering urge in his prettily masculine soul. He'd "force" her to suck him, to serve him, to kneel before him and worship him—calling out terms of abuse they'd both agreed on in platonic moments, where they, ever equals, planned scenarios of her rape-fantasies, her ravishment-fantasies, her slavery-fantasies, she gently encouraging him to open up to his own darkness, his own beautiful uglinesses, in a way he'd never imagine doing in reality. They played at dark parodies of their backgrounds, various revenge fantasies of him as a dirty, angry poor boy from the wrong side of the canal, and she a pampered, privileged princess who he forces to serve him, abducting her and making her pay for all her hauteur. He'd beat her with leather thongs and with rubber whips, forcing her to kiss the flails, to smell them and suck them, to kiss his hands and feet and lick the dirt off his skin. Lately, just lately though, he'd asked if she could take the converse role with him, if he could be punished for his boorish ugliness, which, feigned as it was, was a fetish both of them played with in order to sublimate the real differences in their genders, in their origins. He, too, felt the thrill of the bottom, a dirty pig to be slapped and teased and humiliated, made to wear humiliating makeshift harnesses of rubber strips and leather strips tied tight enough to make his hard pinkish parts come purple and limp, crawling in the mud at her feet, as she, for the first time in her love life, allowed her own urges to dominate, to humiliate and control and punish, to well up from her own unacknowledged depths, to know what Johanna had long known with her. They played at "flipping" one another, as Katharina had done professionally, but only just now for pleasure, and this pretty power game was one that adorned all that was basic and natural in their lusts for one another. They made love for hours in these ways, the daylight through the dirty window glass fading to darkest greys before it all ended. But, it ended, as it had to end, and she lay with him on the great canopy bed in his arms, realizing again that life was a bore and a tragedy, that all solace was fleeting.

Theodor was attuned to Katharina's emotions. He had a

natural sense of empathy and compassion for people in distress, and he sensed correctly that his lover was in a bad state. He knew enough not to try to "cheer up" his friend; instead, he lay there, silent, stroking her raven hair, long grown out of its pink, waiting for her to open up.

"I'm not really mad at Johanna," she said at length. "I just . . . I just wish things weren't so fucking ephemeral. Y'know?"

Theodor nodded.

Then, Katharina realized she was not the only person in the universe, that her burdens were rather light in comparison to others—to Theo's, for instance. How was he to make a living, now? Was he okay?

"Sure," he said, though he was not certain at all. He'd have to go on relief, to be at the mercy of such bureaucrats as Johanna made a living torturing. He was scared. She sensed this, as well as the falseness of his front of joviality, which she knew was partially for her benefit, partially from his own acculturation as a proletarian male. He did not show his feelings much. Or at least, he tried not to.

"How's your Papa?" she asked.

Theodor shook his head.

"I ain't told him yet," he said. "I'm sure he'll be rather disappointed in me. . . . I wish to Christ he wasn't such a fucking Social Democrat."

Katharina did not understand.

"Well," he told her, "he still accepts the rule of the bourgeoisie, and figures that when you get fired, there's something you did to deserve it. He's such a contradiction! I mean, on the one hand, he remembers the glory days, the old days, the heroic time when Otto Bismarck put his kind in jail, and he had to fight. And then, in the same breath, he apologizes for the whole capitalist mess, and thinks he might have, in another time, another place, become a millionaire, if he'd only worked 'hard enough.' It's so weird, Katharina."

Then, out of nowhere, Theodor brightened.

"You wanna meet 'im???" he smiled.

Katharina looked at him, and coughed a surprised chuckle.

"Why, sure," she said. "When?"

"How 'bout right now??"

"Now?"

"Sure! I mean, if I bring over a nice girl, he might be

inclined not to be so awful when I spring the news on him. I mean, about having no money, no prospects, and the fact that we'll both soon be in the gutter."

Katharina wanted to say something. She wanted to say that, as long as she was around, Theodor need never fear being thrown out into the street. But, she didn't say this. Instead, she got her clothes together, and followed him out into the evening.

Theodor's Papa was not at his flat when they arrived. This meant one thing. He'd gone to the beer hall, to be with his buddies. The beer hall was a five-story building, deep in the heart of the industrial district, a place run by and for loyalists of the Social Democracy. From there, a generation ago, great plans had been hatched for the replacing of capitalism with a workers' republic. That those plans had never materialized meant little to the folks who still drank there. It was a kind, old place, of long oak tables scratched with initials of old comrades who had passed into the socialist, atheist afterlife, of barrels of dozens of brands of good beer, of old men singing in their cups songs of not-yet-dashed hope, of generous windows and busty, smiling middle-aged barmaids, lazy, hazy now, its once fevered activity long a memory. Old workers gathered there, now, to drink dreams of past glory and the comforts of working class conformity. It was a place just right for Theodor's father.

Katharina was one of the few girls in the place, and the old men eyed her with a mix of suspicion and grudging attraction that she found very funny. Theodor himself was known here, as the little boy of Ricard Priser, who had stood up on tables and sung revolutionary songs at the age of three, all at his father's urgings and encouragement. Theodor's first pilsner was drunk here, his first lager and ale and porter and stout but a few years thereafter. And the first time he'd been really drunk was at an Oktoberfest celebration when he was thirteen, in these same smoky halls. Theodor knew the old workers, smiled and laughed with them, all friendly like, even though in his heart he thought them all dinosaurs. The real Revolution was not to be found in these beer gardens, in these wide and dimly lit beery halls. The real Revolution was something that might well line up all these stodgy old men against a wall someday.

Theodor's Papa sat at a table with some old comrades, among whom was Theodor's "uncle," a corpulent seventy-year-old plumber named Gustav Cole, who had changed his surname from Cohen when he was twelve because he as a kid in a Catholic part of town was tired of being beaten up everyday by gentiles. They were drinking Belgian Witt from a pitcher, a little apart from the other old men, and had imbibed enough that their eyes were heavy and their countenances gay. They were talking of old times.

"Hey, Vati."

The old man twisted round, regarding his son with a smile.

"Hey, there, Theodor, son. Who's yer friend?"

"This is Katharina."

"Hi!" said Katharina. She was a bit nervous.

Uncle Gustav hailed them both warmly.

"Your Vati and I were just talking about Saxony."

"Yeah," Theodor said. "It's an . . . interesting situation."

Saxony was a province in the throws of a worker's revolt. The Communists there had formed a coalition breakaway government with the left wing of the SPD, and that had stirred up a lot of interest among this old guard this fall: Could the Communists be trusted? Would the alliance bring them all into the fold of some once-regaled unified front? Would the Weimar government march against the workers in Saxony, bringing on another civil war? And would the Russians march across Poland to defend the new, soviet-style republic?

Theodor was not averse to such discussions; indeed, he'd been championing the talk on the subject during his last days of work, more outspoken about it than even his other Spartakist comrades. (This was probably why he'd been fired.) But, he knew the limitations of such talk, with his father and his father's old friend, and all the other old men in the musty beer hall. Theory was great, and action greater. But propriety, and safety, trumped such things. No converts, on either side, would be made today.

Theodor sat down with Katharina at his side. They were poured some beer, and drank it with growing ease in the old men's welcome. Papa Priser was warm, but less interested in his son. He was much more taken with Katharina, whom he decided right then and there to call "Käthe." She smiled at the diminutive.

"So, Käthe, what do you think of the crisis?"

"You mean Saxony, Herr Priser?"

Papa Priser smiled grandly, a little drunkenly, and told her, "'Herr Priser' was my father's name, Käthe. You call me Ricard."

Katharina smiled.

"Well, Ricard, I think the rising up of workers is a good thing. I don't really trust the parties to do anything for them, though."

"You think Russia will invade?"

"I think it doesn't really matter. If the workers are successful, then they won't need the Russians. And, anyway, why would Russia help? They don't want the workers in power. It'd make their own workers get uppity again, like before the bureaucrats killed the Revolution back when they massacred the Kronstadt sailors in '21."

This made Papa Priser's eyebrows knit. He looked to his son.

"Your fraulein's a pretty smart cookie, there, Theodor," he said.

The father and the son had argued this point, and many similar points, a lot over the past days. Theodor, of course, hoped for a Russian invasion; his Papa hoped against it. But, always, the issues were quite clear—workers' power, or not. Had the workers not gotten enough already? Could there ever really be a truly Socialist world? Could people ever really be that good to one another? Were we as human creatures hard-wired to Power—an evil surely—but perhaps one necessary to the continuance of civilisation? These were the issues the father and the son wrangled over. It was refreshing to have somebody in their intimacy who simultaneously agreed with both of them, and neither. It made Papa Priser muse on this new girlfriend of his son, wondering about her, till all at once he connected.

"Ah!" he said in sudden revelation—"So, Käthe, you're the 'anarchist' my liebschin's been telling me about!"

Katharina smiled, realizing the labelling was not accusation.

"I am an anarchist, Herr Priser. Yes, I am."

"Again, Käthe, dear, my name is Ricard. If you're an anarchist, I'm sure you don't need to bother with such proprieties as 'Herr' anybody."

"I remember the anarchists," Uncle Gustav said dreamily, scratching the long scar, dark brown against his light brown face, that had not quite healed since fascists attacked him two years back. "Back in the days of the International—the *First* International, mind. Actually knew a few of 'em pretty well. Good people. A little *crazy*, but good. They fought for the unions as hard as any of 'em."

Katharina didn't say anything, just smiled. "Crazy" was not an entirely bad word to her. And the feeling was one of fellowship, of *Gemutlichkeit*. She liked the company of these old men. But, inevitably, there came questions which were not so easy, not so cosy. Theodor's father asked Katharina what her parents did for wages.

"My . . . parents?" she said, stalling, and Theodor came to her defence with an odd non-sequitur.

"Käthe's family's Jewish, Papa," he said.

The eyes of the elder Priser widened again.

"Oh, yeah?"

Katharina looked at Theodor, then at his father, and said, a little defensively, "That's right."

To see Theodor's father's face brighten, it was as if he'd just been told Katharina was Karl Marx's own grand niece. Katharina did not understand it, and was slightly uncomfortable for a moment; but it was as if, in a world without royalty, she'd been suddenly afforded in the elder Priser's eyes a mark of nobility. He asked her several questions, gentle questions, about her origins, her schooling, her religious philosophy, and then told her that he'd been raised by a Jewish family, who looked after him when his mother, a single woman, had been away at one of her three jobs she worked to keep him out of an orphanage. He told her, with some pride, but mostly humble wonder, that the family had actually asked him to convert as a boy, and that he'd almost agreed.

Katharina found this all a little strange, but not in an unpleasant way. She was used to her Jewish origins being a barrier between herself and the rest of the world. Prejudice was high in Germany, as in all Europe, as in all the world. But Papa Priser seemed almost to take the reverse attitude of most of the gentiles she'd known. He was impressed by her, as if she somehow was personally responsible for the wealth of scholarship, art, and culture he credited Jewish people with giving the world over the centuries, and she didn't have the heart to tell him that she'd rejected her religion almost entirely over her years, that she viewed the whole concept of Judaism through the lenses of Bakunin's *God and the State*—a religion, as all religions, that were part of the problem with the world. Only Eros did she worship any more, and that was a force too divine for deity; only drunken, steamy fucking could get you into Her trances, could let you read the words of His unwritten gospel, penned in sweat and blood and the charged elixirs of yours and your lovers' hot, delicious fluids. A thousand miles away, such worship from this familial scene! But it was quaint, this almost-worship of her bloodline, the "covenants" her ancestors had supposedly made with far-less-sexy spectres, that the old man, an atheist-socialist, weirdly reverenced. She decided that she liked Papa Priser, even though she rather felt that prejudice for something was not too dissimilar from prejudice against it.

Working class people dealt in prejudices, she thought then, or rather, they dealt in *feelings*. Sentiments. It was quite impossible to be neutral about anything. You either felt strongly hate, or strongly love. And after all, love was love, however unrefined the expression of it was. Yes. She liked Papa Priser. And she understood what Theodor had done in bringing all this up: she had not been "outed" as a member of the hated class that even the union bureaucrats of the right wing of the Social Democracy railed against. By the time they parted company, Theodor's father had completely forgotten his curiosity about Katharina's class background. He'd found something much more salient to occupy his heart.

"You stay out just as long as you like, son," said Theodor's Papa as they left, goodly tipsy, from the Social Democrat beer hall an hour later. "Stay out till tomorrow, if ya like. I'll be fine here with Uncle Gustav . . ."

Theodor was happy as he walked with Katharina out of the beer hall into the street. And Katharina was happy, too. She'd met the old man, finally, and the meeting had been better than she could have imagined. It was not too much of a stretch to say that the old man loved her now. And Theodor had not had to deal with his father's disapproval, which still held him fast, like some kraken of the deep, dragging him down into the depths. No. He was in his father's good graces, entirely. He was dating a good girl. He wondered aloud when his father would ask them when they'd marry.

"Marriage?" laughed Katharina.

Theodor smiled.

"It'll come up, I'm sure."

"Well, brother . . . what do *you* think about it?"

Theodor pinched his face in thought.

"I dunno," he said. "I dunno if I really wanna get married—I mean, at least not soon. I mean, do you?"

Katharina laughed.

"Hell no!" she declared. "I don't wanna be property, Theo!"

"Yeah . . . yeah, I guess I don't wanna own each other, neither."

They walked on, into the dark dawn of the newborn evening, moonless on the spottily lamp-lit streets, the wintry wind blowing the last of the autumn leaves along with the trash into chilly spirals along the gutter. Theodor smiled.

"Käthe," he said.

"What?"

"Käthe. It's a pretty name my father called you."

Katharina squinted in mild displeasure.

"I don't really like 'Käthe.'"

"Huh. Well, love, I need to call you something. Something endearing, y'know? Like you call me 'Theo.'"

A look came into Katharina's face, an impish, almost naughty look.

"Katya," she said, smiling.

"Katya?"

"Yeah, Theo. You should call me 'Katya.'"

"That's good. Brings out your Russian sympathies."

"Well, modern anarchism *did* start in Russia."

"So it did."

"D'you like it, baby?"

"Katya? Yeah, sister. I could get into calling you that. It's . . . *sexy.*"

She smiled, and hugged him, pecking him on the cheek. Then they walked, hand in hand, reflecting on their changed names, as well as their changed relationship. They were in Theo's father's eyes now practically engaged. They thought on this, both aloud and to themselves, trudging past a boarded-up shop plastered with posters of old flicks mingling with newer spreads of Socialist, Communist, and Nazi propaganda. Somebody had scrawled an arrow between the bald spectre of last year's "Nosferatu" and a recent iconic rendering of the balding Lenin. Theo couldn't help but chuckle unwillingly at the parallel, though most of his mind was on the beautiful woman with her hand in his, squeezing tight. Silently, they thought of themselves as really together, for the first time. And they knew they were together in the unique way they both wanted to be together—not monogamous, not "tied" in any way. They knew, with the feeling of profound commitment, that they would never,

ever marry. And that bonded them as closely as two lovers could ever be.

By the time they got back to Katharina's flat, others had arrived for the nightly festivities. Johanna was there.

"So, where the hell have you been?" Johanna demanded, as if mocking the question that would erupt from Katharina's own lips, had she not.

Katharina just laughed. She didn't want to make a scene, not in front of all their friends.

Johanna answered her own question. She'd found an apartment on the West End, near the Spandau neighbourhood by the Spree, much more fashionable than this place, much better for business. That Prussian bureaucrat had bought her a mink coat. And there were others, too, who were bringing her presents nightly. Things were good for Johanna, and Katharina was pleased to hear it all, forgetting all about the ire and hurt she'd carried all week. Then, Johanna took Katharina aside, and whispered a question in her ear, glancing curiously at Theodor.

Katharina smiled.

"No," she said. "Theo's still a virgin, that way."

"Well!" Johanna said, a little louder than necessary—"We'll just hafta see what we can do about *that!*"

Before Theodor knew what was happening, Johanna and Katharina, with the conspiratorial laughter of naughty schoolgirls, had taken him by the hand and led him out of the apartment, back onto the street. Where were they going?

To a Blue Moon . . .

Chapter 6

A Blue Moon was cramped and smoky. It was little more than a cellar, down a flight of steps from a shadowy side street, a few blocks away from the flat, easily missed by passers-by, almost a speakeasy in flavour. It was a place for people in the know, one of a hundred and sixty such places in Berlin, queer bars, transvestite bars, lesbian and gay-boy and many other variations on the "inverted" theme—including more than a few which were little more than galleries—*zoos*—where the queer and crazy put themselves on display for adventuresome straight Berliners and tourists indulging their morbid curiosity. This place was far from the beaten path, far from such ménageries; a reference point in the yet underground culture, a convergence of faggots from all over Germany and well beyond, a place that had been there back before the War, before many of those hundred-sixty places even existed— part of an old joke that took the tongues of shameless queens who hung onto discretion from necessity, yet with the boastful effeminacy that underlay the whole scene—*"I meet a man, every once in a Blue Moon . . ."*

After much half-whispered talk and gaudy rumours, Theo found the place much as he'd thought it would be, garish and understated, all at once. Not an upscale place, like the nearby Alexander-Palast; more a dive, like that dyke bar, Taverne, further on, or the Adonis-Lounge across the canal. Downscale, yet cheery, too—"Like the Adonis might be," Johanna said, "if they'd open a window every once in a while, and let the sunshine in. . . ."

Like that rough pick-up joint, the Adonis (or "the Pits," as many called it), a Blue Moon had windows that you couldn't open, painted over in black to disguise it from both Bullen and bullies who might pass by, and sunlight would be hard to picture ever entering the rathskeller. But little gaslights burned low but steady along the walls between columns (which were but glorified studs in the wall), walls painted in Chinese Imperial vermilion, dulled with age and years of smoke, the floral patterns long since lost. Paintings hung on the walls, amateurish canvases of naked and orgiastic scenes reminiscent of Hieronymus Bosch, vaguely foreboding, but somehow celebratory also. Though amateurish in style and talent, these paintings seemed treasured by the proprietors, who endowed them with rich gilded frames, inches thick, that together with the gloom made them seem quite fine indeed. The furnishings in the place had the same baroque elegance, neither understated nor ornamental, like the stock of a furniture shop owing its inventory to down-on-their-luck petty-bourgeois dowagers, who'd stuffed a lifetime of living into their shabby rooms and had to let a lot of it go in shivering anticipation of their demise. Oak and ebony, pine and cherry wood, cedar and mahogany, the armchairs and divans surrounded the little round tables in a mismatched unity, too eclectic to impress, yet pleasing in that no obvious effort was being made *to* impress. Mostly it was all a backdrop; the real drama was the patrons.

Men, dandied or butch, young or older, a mix of styles in which Theo was content in his grey overalls and black leather commie cap, as Katya and Johanna were in their more garish, girlish styles.

"You'll find the boys'll like you," Katya assured as they found a little table. "You're that 'rough trade,' 'butcher' look that drives the old queens wild."

Theo chuckled. He'd never thought of himself as a "type." Indeed, it seemed a little odd to find his whole working class demeanour, his dress, origins, politics, and all, becoming a kind of fetish. He did not think of himself as particularly "rough," or even particularly masculine, however much he'd played at parodies of it with Katya in their times together. But Katya saw it all quite clearly in him now. She liked him for it, though she saw his nascent, burgeoning femme side, too, in the tone of his voice at certain times, in the elegant cast of his visage. His eyes. They were warmer, softer than his style, a shimmering darkness to contrast with his pallor and his sandy hair, and Johanna especially toyed with the idea of Theo in a dress, or as Katya teased, a skirt—short, modern, slutty. Make-up, too, especially dark liner round his eyes, would be perfect. And a corset, Johanna smiled evilly, pulled just a little *too tight.* Theo did not object, smiling almost coyly at his girlfriends; he just felt it best to take his metamorphosis in baby steps.

The three all squeezed onto a curving divan alcoving into a wall, leaving two spinning armchairs vacant in front of them. They didn't stay vacant long.

A pale old queen and his dark lover, a "Rhineland Bastard" as the Nazis called them—part German, part Senegalese—though this teenager was at least a decade older than that child's generation would be—maybe a Senegal soldier who'd stayed around after the occupation of the Rhineland after the War—or his younger brother, enticed by lurid tales, coming to drink in the sights and pleasures of the gloriously tawdry metropolis—invited themselves to sit down at the table. The young black fellow, slight and near silent and sulky, spent his time rolling a cigarette, which seemed more than a cigarette, whilst the old queen parleyed cattily with Johanna and Katya who, though girls, were well-known here. They seemed old acquaintances, though curiously, no names were exchanged, and to Theo no introductions were made. Theo's eyes dwelt a while on the black boy's down-turned face, though the interest appeared anything but mutual. The older man seemed also completely uninterested in Theo, though not unaware. He seemed to be weighing the case of this young butch yet pretty fellow out of the corner of his eye, even as he chatted flamboyantly with the girls in cheeky rumours and innuendos about mutual acquaintances.

Theo decided he was getting a little bored with it all. He did not fit in here, he thought, a little cynically. People probably viewed him as some straight fellow, uninteresting, perhaps even ugly, according to their obscure beauty standard. This feeling of not fitting in was fast becoming an almost physical sensation of disappointment, embarrassment, coupled with a shade of inadequacy—even a twinge of self-loathing. Where *did* Theo fit in? If not here, then *where?*

Where indeed? Trying to mask his disappointment, he got up and crossed the narrow floor of closely dancing men to the bathroom, where he found a urinal and stood there a moment perfunctorily, without really needing to go. He went to the basin and washed his hands, regarding his face. He was, after all, attractive; he knew that. But his ruggedness, his masculine, proletarian, almost peasant bearing, made him feel a little like a fraud here. Would he like himself, had he been another man?

No. He would not.

Sighing, resigning himself to a rather boring and disappointing night, he began to turn away from his mirror reflection, his last glance falling on the red star of his cap, a curious inspiration which he felt sure nobody here would understand, but which filled him with renewed purpose. At exactly that moment, he heard a voice he half-thought his own, saying *"Spartakist."*

It took Theodor a second to realize the voice was not his own. It belonged to another fellow, in the mirror beside him, who had just stepped unseen from a water-closet stall.

Theodor looked at the pretty, dark fellow, with slickly curly black hair, short but a little wild, in a cheap but fine beige tweed suit fitting him as if tailored for him special, but from its quality could not have been anything but off-the-rack. His face was a trim black goatee, dark, dark eyes, framed in consciously archaic pince-nez spectacles, and a smile so warm that Theodor realized his naming him was anything but derogatory.

"Yes," Theodor said. "I am."

The fellow smiled, and offered his hand.

"Guaril," he said. "I'm a big fan."

Theodor chuckled. He took the hand. The shake was neither firm, nor limp. It was, rather, *warm*. Theodor felt he could feel the fellow's blood coursing through his fingers.

"Theodor," he said, then corrected, "Theo."

"Theo. Glad to meet you. This is your first time here?"

Theo smiled.

"That obvious, huh?"

"Yes. You're not dressed really right for the place. But, that's part of the reason I wanted to talk to you."

"You wanted to talk to *me?*"

"Yes. See, I have been in town for about a month, now. You can tell my German's a little off, no?"

"Oh, I think you're doin' just fine there, brother."

Guaril smiled.

"Kind," he said. "You're a kind soul, aren't you, Theo?"

Theo chuckled.

"Kind," he continued, "to be here, dressed like that, and to be a Spartakist."

"What else would I be?"

"You're not just interested in 'workers,' no? You're also interested in *people*. That's *why* you're a Spartakist."

Theo looked at him, grateful, but ignorant, of his drift.

"I'm a Rom, brother," Guaril said. "You know this term? I'm a *Gypsy*."

"Huh."

"I could tell by looking at you, out there in the bar, from the corner where I noticed you, that you would understand that. You know? To be an *outsider*, yes? That's what you were feeling just now, looking at yourself in the mirror. You were feeling that you don't belong in here. Yet, you came here because you didn't belong out there, either. A hard place to be . . ."

Theo looked into Guaril's eyes, deeply, trying to construe

his meaning, his intent. Was he hitting on him? Is this what fags talked about when they were hitting on you? Or, was this a case of something more real (it certainly *felt* more real): was this the beginning of a friendship?

"So," Theo smiled, a little slickly, but also sincerely, "you're attracted to the company of outsiders, then?"

The warm eyes smiled.

"Very," he said.

They looked at each other in the pregnant pause which followed; then, still looking, still smiling, they began to laugh. Theo clapped his hand on the fellow's arm, and said, "C'mon, brother—lemme buy ya a drink."

Guaril clapped his hand on Theo's arm, and said, "Thanks—I'd love a drink."

They walked back out, into the crowd, to find the young black boy and the old white one had left the table, where Johanna and Katharina (*Katya*, Theo remembered) were talking in giggly whispers. Theo and Guaril sat down on the swivel armchairs, Theo proudly introducing his new friend to his old ones.

Katya smiled coyly at Theo, approving, then glanced to Guaril, and touched his hand in welcome. Johanna smiled, also proudly, as if she were responsible for the pairing of the two boys, concluding already that the two were meant for her bedroom (either her new digs or her old—with herself discretely drinking with Katya in whichever parlour). Oh, yes, she said with her eyes, looking over her three companions as if they were all her protégés, *yes, you shall all soon learn the joys of true love . . .*

They drank and chatted, getting along wonderfully over the next hour or so. Johanna drank some mixed things of vodka and gin, Katya some straight shots of cheap Kentucky bootleg bourbon, Theo crisp pilsners in tall steins, Guaril a single glass of Jamaican rum. Guaril nursed his glass the whole hour, gladly putting in his share for other rounds, but politely declining any refreshment. Theo wondered why he drank so little. As the beers affected him, he thought to ask him.

"I drink just a little," Guaril smiled winningly, "at a time."

His new friends were anything but such drinkers. They all got very silly, as the rounds went on. Guaril, too, seemed silly. Maybe he just wasn't much of a drinker. Theo couldn't tell if this made the young man seem younger or older in his mind. Was he wiser, more reserved and sober, over a lifetime of experience? Or was he inexperienced, even naïve, alcohol such a new thing that he didn't quite trust it yet?

A little of both, Guaril chuckled at Theo's query. The four of them had left A Blue Moon, all of them stumbling a little on the icy streets, making their way back to Katya's flat. Katya and Johanna were arm-in-arm, whilst Theo and Guaril talked quietly between the ladies' giggles. Both couples were in on some separate but related private jokes with each other, though exactly what the nature of it all was was obscure. It had something to do, everyone realized, with what they'd all do when they got back home.

Though they had talked at length back in the bar, nobody really knew much about the others from their conversation. They'd parleyed jokes and small talk and witty, catty remarks about how un-hep the *burgerlich* outside world was to whatever they all thought of themselves. And this had a certain currency, this talk, for the world outside their circles was both cold and, frankly, odd, at least in relation to what the four themselves thought of as right and normal. Johanna had been up front about being a prostitute, and had regaled them all with funny tales of clients she'd had, and their queerest fetishes. She especially liked linking the kinkiness of particular men to the straight jobs they had in the world, and marvelling at the apparent contrasts. Katya had briefly made a jest about Theo's red star, taking his cap and putting it on each of the party's heads, before finally returning it to his own. But, aside from saying something unintelligible about "dialectics" and its relation to something (she was laughing a lot, and Johanna kept interrupting), there was nothing political at all about their conversation. Theo missed that. For, he'd originally been attracted to Guaril because of his comment about Spartakism, or rather his sentiment about it, and he'd have loved to get into something more substantive, just because he liked talking about such things. Guaril, after all, could become his comrade someday—or perhaps he already was—but, even if only a sympathizer, it was something to talk about the burning issues of the day, and even theory, with somebody new.

When they got back to Katya's flat, the jazz combo downstairs was playing so loud it could be heard even through the heavy door, and certainly through the floor which positively shook with the snares and the high-hats, the strums of banjos and the rumbling, stand-up bass. They were playing something between Paris and New Orleans, something very good, the horns and violins making sweet love in their entwining solos, so the foursome didn't mind listening to its muffled but pulsing serenade in the night. Johanna took Guaril by the arm, unexpectedly, and drew him to her once-again chamber, with the disarming enticements of a skilled diplomat. Why she'd taken him aside was a mystery; but it afforded Katya and Theo a chance to talk.

"You *like* him, don't ya?" she laughed in a whisper to Theo, who was helping himself to some red wine from the parlour cabinet. He couldn't help giggling a little.

"You think so, huh?" he teased.

"Oh, yeah. Yeah, liebling, you *want* that boy."

"Yeah, but does he want me?"

"Well, love, he *did* come back with you from the bathroom. That's *always* a good sign."

Theo took a second to realize the innuendo. He laughed out loud.

"We didn't *do* anything!" he protested. "We just . . . *met* there."

"Oh, yes, darling—I meet some of my *best* bosom pals in the bathrooms of pansy bars."

Theo looked to Katya, and could tell by her smile and manner that there was no need to ask the next question. But, he asked it anyway.

"Do you mind?" he said.

"You two?" she said. "Why on *earth* would I mind that?!"

Theo sighed, all measure of confidence returning to him.

"Just thought I'd ask, schätzele," he said. "I think I *ought* to ask."

"Well, sure, Theo. In the future, I guess it would be good to ask. But, you know about me and Johanna. And now, you've got Guaril. Everything's smooth as silk."

"Well, what about other people? Should we ask? Or, should we just do what we do, and talk about it later? Or, should we, maybe, *not* talk about it?"

Katya lost her smile.

"No, love," she said, "I don't ever think we should *not* talk about it. No, never that. That's what boring married people do to each other, when they're cheating. You and I aren't cheating. We *can't* cheat—unless, we lie. Or, try to hurt each other."

"I'd never try to hurt you, Katharina."

She smiled.

"I know," she said. "My beautiful, beautiful boy—*my*

Theodor."

Johanna called to them, then, her tête-à-tête with Guaril evidently concluded. He was laughing under his breath, trying not to, though she was in good form and control.

"What's so funny?" Theo laughed, echoed by Katya.

"Nothing!" blurted Guaril, a little shamefaced, trying not to giggle.

"Why, nothing, darlings," assured Johanna grandly. "Our new friend here was just telling me some things I needed to know; that's all."

The couple looked to the two with scepticism. But, the hell with it, they thought; let Johanna have another one of her secrets. Guaril, evidently, was being let into some intimacy, and this was to be welcomed. He was a member of the family, now . . .

This was something that became a theme that night. For, what Johanna had talked about with Guaril was something which assumed proportions not even they could have foreseen. She'd asked him how he'd feel about engaging in a ritual, something beyond the one-to-one expression of sexuality Guaril might have anticipated before coming here tonight. Johanna had plans. She got them all high on opium and hashish, imparted tastes of a mixture she kept in one of her handbags she said was called "Satyrin," the golden elixir prepared for Guaril and Theo, the silver for herself and Katya. Then she turned the lights down low.

"Now," she said, with a mind to orchestrate a scene, "you, Theo, want Guaril, don't you?"

Theodor regarded her with resentment at her impertinence. He'd barely talked to Guaril, truth be told, and had not yet thought how he would make his move on the lovely boy. Before he could say anything, Johanna was already talking again, this time to Katya.

"And," she said, smiling, "you, Katya, want Theo."

"Mmm hmm," Katya smiled.

"And, you, Guaril, want both of them."

Guaril got his sweet, shamefaced but happy expression, and sipped his wine.

"Well," pronounced Johanna grandly, "you kids need a proper mummy to tuck you into your common bed. Luckily for you, I am more than experienced in that role. The three of you will find pleasure this eve—but you must do now exactly as *I* say . . ."

The three looked at Johanna with incredulity. But Johanna was not the least bit self-conscious. She'd orchestrated tougher crowds than this, and she was assured of her dominance in matters sexual. She came over, and gave Katya a great, long kiss. Then, piece by piece, she stripped her of her clothing, all of it, till Katya stood naked and voluptuous in the low light.

Directing her without words, Johanna brought her longtime companion, longtime love-slave, to the love seat, and lashed her hands to the wings with the slave's own lacy underwear. She spread her legs apart, and secured them to the love seat's legs with silky scarves that were laying there. Theo and Guaril were silent. Theo wondered at the scene, but found himself turned on, wondering if he were about to be shown another of the scenes between Katya and Johanna he'd been treated to that first night, nearly a year ago in this very room. But, no; there was a different madness to Johanna's method. Guaril was in the know, and smiled in a sweet mix of embarrassment and eagerness. He began to strip himself of his tweed suit, his silky shirt and undergarments, laying them all gingerly and fastidiously on the rocker by the window.

Not understanding, but seeing the general trend, Theo began, too, to disrobe. Johanna came up behind him, and held fast his hands.

"I know you're a randy little *slut,*" she whispered hotly in his ear, *"ain't* ya, Theodor?"

Theo had often thought on Johanna. She was an object of fascination, not simply his own, but of almost everyone in the scene. But never had he allowed himself to really *melt* in her presence, the way he melted now, in the strong, soft grip of her hands, in the hot whispers in his ear. What did she mean to do with him?

Johanna pulled the rest of Theo's clothing off him, almost ripping it from his body—ordering him to stand straight and silent whilst she stripped him. Then, she took his hair and pulled it back, pulling his gaze in the direction of his bound, spread-out lover.

"You *want* her, don't you, little *slut* boy?" Johanna breathed to him. Then, she pulled him to view Guaril, who was standing silent by the window, clothed only in his sculpted, bronze glory.

"And," she breathed, "you want *him*, too—eh *faggot?*"

Theo breathed an almost unwilling breath, a deep grunt of assent. She released his hair, then brought her hand over the round cheeks of his ass, and lingered there, between them.

"Right *here*, little faggot?" she touched his most guarded, most sensitive spot back there, that place he'd thought long and hard about allowing entry, fearing it, yet longing for it, too. She pressed there, feeling it tighten as he winced, then begin to relax with her tiny, massaging circles. "*Right **here**, Theo?" she rasped. "*Look* at that boy, his proud, thick *eight inches*—**longing** for you there. Are you *afraid of it*, Theo?"

Theo felt Johanna's power behind him, felt her strong, soft hands holding his fast, teasing his asshole with just the hint of penetration. For all her fierceness, all her command, she wanted him to yield to her *willingly*. She wanted him to find a hunger down there, knowing from her whispers with Guaril before that he was well aware of what to do with those eight inches, knew well how to romance a boy's virgin ass with all the full and gentle power of a master.

Theo felt a tremor deep inside, felt his legs almost giving way beneath him. *No,* he whispered—he was *not* afraid. Or, rather, he *wanted—**more** than his fear.

"It's just like Katya, Theo," Johanna smiled, pressing in, ever so slightly deeper, "with you. Or even *me,* when I first let in a boy, or the first wondrous fingers of a lady. You have to *open* yourself to it. You have to ***trust . . .***"

The domina took Theo's hands, and secured them fast behind him with a silky tether. Then, she bent him down, over the ottoman, which she kicked over to the love seat's feet. She pushed his face into Katya's cunt, and ordered him to lick her, suck her, fuck her with his tongue. Moaning a high, shivery moan, Theo asked no more questions; he just went to work, tasting and licking, sucking and savouring, whilst Johanna lashed a dog's collar round his neck, which she fastened to a leash that tied round Katya's waist. Thus the bound slave, and the slave's bound slave, began to moan and sigh in perverse and delicious pleasure.

Johanna signalled to Guaril, who knew her will, which was his own. He got behind Theo, and touched his ass like he would a virgin woman's breasts, softly, firmly, smoothing loving circles, in the discovery sweetening a long, patient courtship. He spread Theo's cheeks and pressed up, making him present himself to him. He spat onto his hand, and made circles round the head of his cock, then spat onto Theo's spread out cheeks, over and over, till the spittle trickled down into his wrinkly, puckering skin, and pooled there. Then Guaril eased into Theo's ass, slowly, surely, in one long, driving motion. A full minute it took till the shaft had disappeared into they boy's creamy backside, but never was Guaril not in motion. He leaned his whole body into Theo, kneeling down to thrust into him more fully, his strong, callused hands gripping his thighs. Theo found himself instantly wedded to the feeling of the long cock inside him—the fullness, the vulnerability, the completeness, the power inside him that made him feel exulted, his own cock swelling in delicious agony till it began to pulse in time with the cock inside him, spilling pearls of semen heat onto the floor. Johanna bound Guaril's waist to Theo's, making of his hungry, sumptuous fucking yet another slavery, a slavery which pleased all three. Katya looked down at her lover, beautifully serving her, being fucked by another, who was in that moment also her lover, and felt a wave of rapture rising to engulf her consciousness as the wet pleasure of his frenzied tongue and the vibrations of his groaning combined with the thrusting of Guaril's slow and certain cock, making of the bound boy a channel, a humming, surging conduit of energy.

Johanna had stripped down to her underwear, a tantalizing ensemble of garters and lace, and brought out her best riding crop. She traced the tip of the riding crop along her three protégés' bodies, teasing their flesh, which had blended into one. She struck Katya, once hard, then softly, rapidly, building up quickly to a rapid-fire, punishing the very tips of her breasts, bringing the pinkish-amber nipples gradually to purple bruises. She dallied between that and punishing Theo, who was lost between thrusting and wallowing, his face engulfed and his ass reamed, all slow and steady and hot and frenzied, Johanna spanking his white ass viciously and viciously beating his back, raising pink and red and purplish welts like cuneiform, like hieroglyphs of her own lost love-language. She knew Theodor had always wanted this, had been tickled as he'd almost begged her for it so many times before. She enjoyed the punishing as surely as he'd longed for the punishment, feeling as one with the riding crop as it whistled through the air, her breaths sharp with the rasps of its lashes, jolts of pleasure like lightning through her own moistening cunt hidden beneath her silky underwear—every slash, every slap making her giggle and groan. She beat Guaril just as cruelly, too, his ass rippling with pumping his boy, tightening against the sting of the lash, pumping harder and faster with each of her strokes, plunging deeper into his boy's sweet, wet heat to avoid the stings—Johanna cackling triumphant as his grimace finally melted into a groaning grin as he surrendered to the wedding of pleasure and pain, thrusting his ass out at last to receive her cruelties in *joy.*

For a long, long time, they fucked thus, slaves to their pleasure, slaves to Johanna's triumphant perversity. It was for all of them more than they'd anticipated in the dizzy pansy bar. None of the three protégés had ever been involved in a ménage a trios before, had never really thought what this would mean. But Johanna, the skilled, the experienced, the fearless, had recognized the potential they each had in them, the potential they had together. She knew.

This was but the beginning.

Chapter 7

It was not until the next morning that the threesome really got to know one another. They left the flat in the mildly hungover dawn, hearing the echoes of the jazz combo that had serenaded them in their lustful passions of the night before, a lazy last blast of coronet and violin, too full of joy to heed the end of night; too, they heard a round of cackling from that uncanny, anonymous voice as they traversed the rickety stairs to the street, and they laughed at the laughter, not knowing its meaning in the chill dawn. They went to a little café, some blocks away from the flat, and had early morning porters in the harsh, brilliant light of the late October dawn. Johanna was sleeping off her drinks of the night before (though skilled and in control in the night, she was actually quite drunk, as usual, and had a great hangover awaiting her if she did not take the precaution of sleeping well into the afternoon). This left Katya, Theo, and Guaril to find the early morning streets together, leaving their footprints in the thick snow which had fallen in the night.

The café was somewhere between proletarian and petty-bourgeois—in other words, bohemian, with collages and montages and experimental photographs on the walls by artists known and artists obscure, all of them underground and deliciously, decadently modern. The first substantive thing that was said among the three of them was a comment Guaril made about the art, saying he was interested in doing collage himself.

"Really?" Katya said, interested.

"Yes," said Guaril, a little dreamily. "Collage is my medium. Though painting and etchings appeal to me also. I am a great admirer of John Heartfield and Hannah Höch, among others. Raoul Hausmann and George Grosz, also, though I am less, well—less *ugly* than they are, I hope. Really, I'm trying to find my own way. Don't want to copy them, but, as a beginner, I tend to do that a little. Maybe more than I'm comfortable, yes?"

"I'd love to see some of your work sometime," Katya smiled.

"Yeah," Theo concurred. "I think art is a great way to motivate people."

"Yes," Guaril said. "I believe this, too."

Katya was a little nonplussed by this. She did not think art was there strictly and simply to "motivate" people. She felt that it was a question of finding beauty in life, even in life's ugliness.

That's what she liked about Höch, particularly. Theo took the opportunity to say a little of what Leon Trotsky had had to say about art, that it, along with all cultural forms and institutions, could not be separated from the class struggle going on in a given society. There was no such thing as "apolitical" art. Just as there was no real way to be apolitical about anything. You either sided with the rising revolutionary classes, or you opposed them.

"That's miserably reductionist, I think," Katya said.

Theo shrugged.

"I dunno, suβe," he said. "Just seems like common sense to me."

Katya then said that art could be beautiful, even when it served the interests of the most horrendous and oppressive class systems. The Sistine Chapel, for instance, which she'd seen more than once, visiting it in her youth with her mother and then with her great aunt on holidays to Italy, was the product of feudal Church tyranny, father of countless witch burnings and inquisitions and children's crusades. Yet, to her, it was the most beautiful art in the world.

Theo didn't say anything, though he did not like this. But Guaril conceded her point, as well as affirming Theo's, by saying that Beauty was a product of human beings—workers, essentially, always. Who employed them was irrelevant. Yet, art *could* have a mission, especially in this Modern Era, to advance the cause of enlightenment, and enlightenment in this era was political enlightenment.

Katya continued to object, that art could not be so easily reduced, and that art was not really "pure" if it was simply pamphleteering. Theo got a little hot, then, saying that, to him, Beauty had everything to do with Struggle. The monsters that ran the world were not interested in art for its transformative powers; rather, they were into it because it could be bought and sold, *controlled*, and thus it was *the rulers* who really "reduced" art—by prostituting and blaspheming its power.

"Blasphemy?" Katya smiled. "That's a queer word for a Communist to use."

Theo chuckled.

"I'm an individual, Katya," he said. "I don't just parrot what the Party has to say about something. I *feel* my politics, which are in line with the Bolshevik dream at the moment—but I reserve the right to approach it all according to my own queer, crazy perspective."

Katya reached over and pecked him on the cheek.

"Yes, liebling," she laughed—"and that's why I love you."

Guaril detected the difference between his two lovers, and was curious. If Katya was not a Bolshevik, then what was she?

Anarchism and Communism parleyed for the next ten minutes, not disagreeably, over the porters at the little round table. Guaril listened, weighed, judged. He told them he was not of either ilk. To him, the question was colonialism, European domination of the globe. This was where his political sympathies lay, with the darker peoples of the planet, whom, he said, would one day arise.

"Look at Nazism," he said, no longer dreamy, sharp rather. "All it is is European domination turned inward. Whiteness, as a political concept, has evolved over the centuries, in order to justify the expansionism of European rulers—as well as their white subjects. All the Nazis want to do is look inside Europe, and 'purify' the white races within it. Jews, Gypsies, and others who do not 'fit'—these are being targeted as simply the logical progression of what the Europeans generally have been doing to black, brown, red, and yellow peoples for centuries."

Theo and Katya nodded. They hadn't really ever considered it that way. But they both opposed colonialism, had wept over the memories of Indians and Aboriginals and Laplanders, had perceived the racist, imperial power dynamic, which they recognized and decried as pure evil in the world today. Neither of them had any illusions about "progress" or even the "evolution" of societies. Theo, by training, had a certain affinity for thinking of civilisations "progressing"; but he always kept in his heart the feeling that what was called "primitive communism" by Marx had everything to do with the correct way of relating to one another in egalitarian community. What was the point, he'd always felt, in pushing the European capitalist misery onto peoples of the planet who had never developed class society in the first place? He recalled well how the Social Democrats, the majority party in many of the parliaments of Europe for years, had justified the cruel colonial projects of their nations in Africa and Asia, arguing that the "primitives" of these places would benefit from the introduction of capitalism into their countries—for how else could they ever evolve into socialist societies, working class power, if they did not first become "workers" in the European, capitalist sense? (This disingenuous misuse of Marxist theory was yet another thing Theo had against the Second International.) It seemed to Theo that the European peoples, rather than having the "civilised answer" the darker races needed, had much to learn from these so-called "primitives," and as Trotsky had recently written, sarcastically but sincerely, answering a polemic thrown at Communists by a racist pamphleteer, and quoting what that bastard had spat against the morality of the Communists, Theo would rather stand with "the morality of the Kaffirs" over any bullshit "superiority" of the white race.

Guaril said he knew a little of anarchism, a little more of communism, but had never really committed himself to either. One thing he admired about Lenin was his position on the self-determination of oppressed nations. This was, in Guaril's eyes, very close to a correct position, and a very enlightened one for a European man to take. Theo smiled. He was proud of Comrade Lenin for that, as he was proud of Engels who had written so poignantly of the Irish Question in the last century, and the need for English tyranny to end with English workers purging themselves of their bigotry. No one who really valued Socialism could entertain racist notions, or their Socialism was not correct. It was simple science, eventually. Racism was worse than simply ugly or wrong; it was an ideology of the ruling class, the enemy class, and it was detrimental to the proletariat's rise to power. It had to be destroyed, violently if necessary, purged from the minds of the proletariat, who had nothing in common with their masters. Otherwise, the proletariat would never succeed in rising.

They talked, then, of matters more personal, which was tied up with the political, as nearly everything was in this highly political time. Katya talked of her origins, her family, and the strangeness of being from the master class and yet siding profoundly with their antithesis. Theo shared his own history, the privation of his family, the kind of drama that underlay everything in the working class, the fiery emotions of his family, who might yell at you, beat you, put onto you impossible demands out of guilty loyalty—but in the end, you knew they loved you, overwhelming you with that emotion, to a degree that was sometimes uncomfortable, assailing your individual sovereignty. Yet, at the end of the day, the love was real, palpable, welcome and comforting. Katya said she admired and envied that love. She herself often wondered whether her parents were truly capable of love, for they thought that expressing strong emotions, of any kind, was somehow in bad taste. She'd never recalled seeing them quarrel, yet she was quite sure they did, and often. Whilst she'd been spared the overturned tables and the flying pots and pans, she also felt that, in the truest sense, she had no idea who her parents really were. Any sincere feelings that may have lain between them had never been spoken, and it was far too late now.

Guaril smiled. To him, these friends represented the extremes of class in the European world. And he envied them both, in his way.

"I was taken away from my family," he told them, smiling as if the tragedy's sting had long gone soft, but still left its scars. "When I was just three or four, the government of Spain took me and my brothers and sisters from my family, and we were all raised apart. I never knew my parents after that. I don't even know where they are. They could be dead. I've lost touch with my siblings, too. I was raised to forget my origins, my culture. Yet, at the same time, the white families and the white schools which raised me never let me forget that I was of the Roma. I was an outsider, from the youngest age. And, now, I feel a stranger to my own people, too. Raised to be a Gadjo, I've drunk the poisonous measure of that Gadjo culture as if it were mother's milk, till I no longer know the taste of my own blood. I am ignorant of my culture, my language, my religion. I am an orphan, twice—thrice over."

Theo and Katya were stunned into silence. What could you say to such a story? What could you feel, but profound sympathy, which no words could ever really express?

Guaril smiled, then. He knew his new friends felt for him, and he intimated that it was amongst his friends that he came closest to feeling that "home" he'd never had. Life was about choices. He'd come to a political consciousness which he'd chosen, as much as simply reacting to what had been forced upon him. He was very proud of his culture, even though he was yet but a poor student of it. He again talked of his solidarity with other darker peoples. He mentioned he'd written to Marcus Garvey, the West Indian African in America who had founded the Universal Negro Improvement Association in 1918. He wanted to know whether there was a chance that he could join.

"What did Garvey say?" Theo asked.

"He wrote me," Guaril said, "very courteously, warmly even. But he said that, whilst he was not at all unsympathetic to me and my plight and my people's struggle—recalling that, like his folk, my people had been enslaved in some parts of the world even into the middle of the 19th Century—noting that, with warmest wishes, Garvey encouraged my organizing, but wrote that with limited resources, he must concentrate his efforts on his own. I understand that. I just wish we Roma could come together like Garvey is doing in Harlem. It'll happen. There's already some stirrings of Roma organizations, here and there, especially in the East. It's simply the course of history, its inevitable evolution to higher and higher consciousness. That's my hope, anyway . . ."

Neither Theo nor Katya put much stock in "race consciousness." For Theo, the self-determination of oppressed nations was a thing to be fought for and defended; but the real task was organizing workers of *all nations*, and he had made this call his own raison d'être, the call to arms against a master class that, too, represented many races and nations. For Katya, the idea of building nations of any kind was suspect. She saw not simply class composition, but the very existence of a nation-state, as the question to be wrestled with. A "workers' state" was a state, same as any other, and as long as it existed, it could only be an enemy to human freedom. If the workers rose up under a red banner, or if the darker peoples of the planet rose up under something more red, black, and green—still, it was flags, still states, and these could never liberate anybody. Katya and Theo again saw their separateness, their difference, and it made them both angry and sad. Neither could embrace the other, on the most profound, most meaningful levels. And that made them wonder about their embrace, on all the levels they could embrace, as potentially fleeting.

They denied this. They laughed, they teased. They did not want it all to end. Especially over something as miserable as politics. And yet, they were both political people, right down to the fibre of their souls. How could they reconcile, when their comrades were sometimes beating each other in the streets?

They were quiet a moment. Theo gulped his porter, as if to drown something he couldn't.

But Guaril, unasked, gave them an answer.

"We," he said, "all of us, are enemies of this order. If the Nazis succeed, and put people in 'segregation' or 'quarantine,' as some of their pamphlets argue for 'undesirables' and 'defectives' of society—but *we* know, both you and I, that they'll put their enemies in those camps soon after the crippled and the retarded and the insane, yes?—if they do this, d'you really think they're going to give much of a damn about what *brand* of reds we are? What *particular colours* our flags are? No, my friends, my comrades. They will put us all in the same cells, and beat us till we shed our common blood, which is red, and human, despite our differences. . . ."

Theo and Katya took unexpected heart from this. It shouldn't be so grim, they both felt. But, in the time they saw coming in Germany, the terrible fights ahead, it really wouldn't matter. They should embrace each other, truly, for their enemy was one, united in their front; their particular differences were washed out in the same, grim White vision. The Nazis and the government did not care a jot for the problems leftists might have in unifying. They hated. And hate was sometimes more salient a bond than love. That was the sad truth. . . .

But Guaril was not despairing. Because, he said, the forces of love in the world always triumphed against the tyrannies of hate, in time. Vlad Dracul had enslaved his people, back in the fourteenth century, when he reigned supreme, almost wiping them from the face of the earth. Surely, then, it must have seemed the monster would succeed. But the Roma people had survived that Wallachian murderer, and now he was long gone and dead and dust—but fodder for penny-dreadful novelettes and cheap flicks about vampires—and meanwhile, Guaril sat here, centuries later, proud and alive.

The thing that welled up in each of their hearts then was an incredible attraction, one that went beyond the merely physical. They were, they began to realize, *Seelengenossen*—that which was the Karmic Quest exhorted for queers by visionary writers in the pages of *Die Freundschaft,* the reason they'd all been reborn in the bodies of intermediate, inverted beings. The quest for the Soul-Mate. *Freundesliebe.* They were *friends*.

And the world was better because of them.

Chapter 8

Old Max was a grounding influence on Theodor, as he was to many of the Spartakists, young and old alike, despite the disagreements he might have had with him over the past years. Max had seen the workers' movement in Germany rise and fall and rise again, his experience extending back into the last century, his knowledge of history and theory something lived, not just read about. And he, unlike Theodor's father, had stayed radical, moving with the times to embrace the Independent Socialists, the Spartakusbund, and even to dalliances with the ultra-left Communist Workers' Party. But one thing he didn't like much, and had no use for, was anarchy.

The Saxon Soviet had risen and collapsed in the last weeks, and it seemed the worker's struggle here in Germany had been gravely set back by its failure to sustain power. In the shadow of that damning event, the comrades here in Berlin moved from talking of practical plans for Germany to theory about workers' politics in general—a retreat, it seemed to Theo, into theory (though he said nothing about it). Old Max talked today on the subject of the Dictatorship of the Proletariat, more in Russia than in Germany or anywhere else, speaking frankly and honestly about some of the Bolsheviks' mistakes, but always with the supportive solidarity of the fellow Party comrade. Theoretical differences were to be more than "tolerated" in the international communist movement. They were to be vigorously encouraged, actually—but always with Comrade Lenin's sensible fighting tactic and policy of "democratic centralism." A comrade was free to disagree with his or her Party, and more, honour-bound to argue for his or her position when he or she thought the dominant one was incorrect. But, whilst the debate was raging within the ranks of the Party, the positions of the organization were to be defended to the outside world, along with the comrades who held them. Old Max was tolerant, but serious. This thing they were doing in the world was not to create an open "talk-shop" of revolution; it was to win a battle, and the forces of the world wanted to destroy not only the physical selves of the workers and the professional revolutionaries who defended them, but the very theoretical strength and unity that made that fight possible.

But this cell meeting was one where Theo expressed his differences with the Party, ones that were beginning to brew in him as a potential revolution all his own. The collapse of Saxony's soviet in just the last days as October had passed into November had left him feeling ornery and frustrated. The old solutions, even if "old" dated only to the last few years since 1917, were beginning to weigh him down in their impracticality, their failure to achieve their stated aims, and even (he was beginning to state in his own mind, though not yet aloud) their hypocrisy. He'd been to Russia once, a guest of the Youth Brigade back in 1918, when the World Revolution had looked so hopeful, so imminent. Revolution had toppled the Kaiser in that year, and a workers' council government had taken over in Austria-Hungary soon after. Communist Parties, in solidarity with the new International, formed almost spontaneously all over Europe in a few scant months, soon thereafter in Turkey, in China—even in far away Indonesia! Theodor had been barely fifteen years old, then. He'd been among the youngest of the emissaries from outside the new soviet workers' republic, thoroughly idealistic, thoroughly dazzled by the things he saw there. He would join the Party proper just a few months after, so won over he was to what he considered the cutting edge of workers' politics, beyond the stodgy socialism of his father, beyond what any other group seemed willing to do. Seeing the soviet system in action, a country where his people, the workers, had actually taken power, had kept him loyal to the German Communists for years after. But, there was something in that visit to Russia that had threatened his idealism, too, things that didn't quite square with the ideal; and its seed once planted had begun, just lately, to germinate. The world-view he'd not challenged back then had become something he could no longer blindly accept. Old Max had been to Russia, too, several times since Theodor. But those things, the things the young, idealistic Theodor found disturbing there, these things were not things that fazed the old comrade. He saw the work the Bolsheviks were doing as the most important work in all the world's workers' struggle. And so, he was willing to cut the Russian comrades a lot of slack.

So were most of the Communists at the cell meeting. They all talked of the coming fight with the fascists, and the need to defend the Revolution against the "social-fascists"—the Social Democrats, who were in every way undermining the work of the Revolution, and were (they affirmed amongst themselves yet again) to be viewed as just as great a threat as the Brownshirts, if not actually worse. The breakaway left-wing Social Democrats had failed in their solidarity with the Communists in the just-overthrown revolutionary council government of Saxony—more than proving to the comrades here their bankruptcy as a party, and the correctness of Moscow's line. There would be no more demonstrations of unity with the SPD.

"What about the anarchists?" Theo said.

"What about them?" Old Max said in stride.

"Well, don't you think it's a good idea to form a kind of bloc with them? An alliance?"

"On what basis, Comrade Theodor? I mean what *theoretical* basis?"

"Easy, Comrade Max. The defence of Revolution. If we cannot count on anyone right of us, surely there's a point to working with those to our left. The Communist Workers' Party, and the United Social Democratic Party—Communists like us, just to our left now. And the syndicalist groups, like the Free Union of German Workers, and the Marine Transport Workers I.W.W.—they've got unions in Bremerhaven, Hamburg, Stettin—maybe other places, too, I'm not sure. Why can't we work with them?—and all the anarchist circles, too, who support workers' revolt? We share something with them."

"What? What do we share? I ask you this because I think you are a good comrade, a good worker and a fine student of theory. But, comrade, I think sometimes you have a little too much—well, for lack of a better term, *faith*—in the potential to work with people outside our Party. You know well the theory; now, let me tell you the practice. Our comrades in Russia have just fought a gruelling civil war with elements of the Old Regime. The White Armies have been finally driven out. But during that civil war, comrade, the ease and freedom which we take for granted here in Deutschland and in other countries outside the Soviet Union was not a luxury they could afford. All the rot about 'repression' that has been perpetrated by our enemies is only the Dictatorship of the Proletariat—the fighting chance we have to save ourselves. It's all well and good to talk about things, to argue. But when you've got a gun to your head, you cannot afford to have a debate with your hands about how to save your head. You've got to have a body that works together. Or, your enemy will kill *everything*. We can make mistakes. But if we don't work together, there'll be no 'we' to make those mistakes.

"The anarchists have been disruptive since they first formed, back when I was younger than you are now. Longer. Marx and Engels had to purge Bakunin and his anarchists from the First International, because of how they would have affected the leadership of the working class. They're dilettantes, comrade. They're petty-bourgeois dreamers—at best! At worst, they march in the armies of the enemy. The uprising of the Kronstadt sailors two years ago was a White insurgency. That's been proven by our comrades consistently and undoubtedly. And it is no government of the working class that does not vigorously and ruthlessly crush such opposition to its existence. This is war, comrade! There is no room for weakness in this hour."

Theo laughed, and shook his head.

"So," he said, "difference of opinion is 'weakness' now, in your eyes?"

"Healthy debate is part of the process. But war is war. And the privates cannot debate the efficacy of the war, if their army is to remain on the battlefield."

"The *privates?* Comrade Max, in the beginning, when Comrade Trotsky organized the Red Army, it was done according to the principle that 'private' and 'officer' was a contradiction inherited from centuries of Czarism. The enlisted men *elected* their officers, the same as they did when they began the Revolution, in the soldiers' councils on the battlefields of the Eastern Front, when they elected to desert the carnage of those fields of death—and *shoot* their warmongering officers!—then march in triumph back to their motherlands. *That* was the Revolution—its very meat, its very substance. Remove that, even for a time, and you've effectively butchered the Revolution. You've killed the spirit in order to impose the letter. And that's no dictatorship of the proletariat. That's the dictatorship of a new class, in the *name* of the proletariat. How is that different from the dictatorship of the bourgeoisie, enacted, say, in the rise of Napoleonic despotism following the fall of the Jacobins?"

The other comrades in the cell were nonplussed by this parallel. Most all of them had had misgivings about some of the recent things the Bolsheviks had done, the outlawing of any other parties besides their own, the militarization of the labour unions, the qualitative change going on in the soviets, the workers' and peasants' councils, which seemed increasingly to be moving from bottom-up expressions of direct democracy, so, so essential to the Revolution when it first started, to top-down organs of Party discipline. But, a new *class?* That was not scientific. It *felt* right;

but it could not *be* right. And Old Max, expert on theory that he was, began to disparage his comrade's lack of theory, his impulsive and reckless assertion that workers' advocates were somehow different in kind than workers at large. What was the *basis— economically*—of such a class? Classes weren't just groups of people; they had to be accounted for, explained, in terms of their relation to the means of production. There was no property any more in Russia. The Revolution had outlawed property, and forcibly appropriated it under the state. Therefore, how could anyone economically dominate?

"I don't know," Theodor admitted. "I don't think there's been anyone who's made a real economic analysis of it. Not yet. But, think about it, Max. Every social phenomenon is a result of class struggle, right? Therefore, there needs to be a social basis for any theory. And, now, the main theorists we have are in a position of power; they have no social need to critique that power."

"So, then," Max chuckled, "you think that there's a social need for criticism from a social class that doesn't even exist? You'll be waiting a while, I think, comrade, for your 'phantom-class' to arise from the ether to explain itself to you!"

"When I went to Russia, comrade, back right after the War, I met workers there, observed the council meetings. These ignorant people, unschooled in anything but struggle, could not see—or rather, they could not *justify*—their own position, to defend their interests against the co-optation of the Party functionaries that were taking over their meetings! The more schooled workers were dominating the less schooled ones! I dunno if that constitutes a *class*, exactly, but there *are* different interests. I could see that even then. Workers' democracy can't be served by limiting democracy. Dialectics aside, something that isn't something just *isn't* something. And any theory that comes out of the Party these days is less interested in really investigating the problem as much as justifying the interests of the Party itself. That's simple materialism, comrade. If there's an anti-worker ideology being propagated, it doesn't matter what class is doing it. It's *anti-worker*, and it'll doom and damn the great experiment going on in the East, as surely as Napoleon and the Directory and the Committee of Public Safety doomed and damned the Great French Revolution, leading to the wars that killed workers and peasants by the *millions!* What I'm trying to say—"

"—What you're trying to say, comrade, is ridiculous! No

wonder you like these anarchists so much! You're practically *one* of them! Think practically, for a moment—get your head out of the clouds! We've got a whole movement to defend—not just in Russia, but all over! It happens that there were reasons for Bonapartism. It secured the class interests of the bourgeoisie, when they did not yet have the political maturity and economic potency to fully rule as a class in their own right. This thing is the same thing. You know where most of the workers who fought the October Revolution are now, comrade? Dead! They're all lost on the battlefields to White Army bullets! They joined the Red Army, and they fought to defend their interests as *only* workers can! Most of the people in the factories now are peasants, fresh from the fields. They have no idea how to proceed with workers' democracy—they don't have enough experience to know how to use their own council system! If you were Comrade Lenin or Comrade Trotsky—what the hell would you do?! Would you let these peasants bring the Czar back?! That's how backward they are, Theodor! Proletarian revolution requires *proletarians*—class-*conscious* proletarians—and most of them are either dead or in the Party. And that's why the Party has to do what it does. To defend the real Revolution against those class elements that seek to destroy it. I don't like draconian measures any more than you do, my young friend, but the problem facing the Party now—the *only party in history* to defend the Revolution as much as they have—in *actual practice*, not just *in theory*—is that their base is dubious, now. What do you do, then? Give up?! Let the reactionaries back into power?! Tell me, young comrade, would *that* be defending the hope of workers' democracy? What if these ignorant peasants got it into their heads to bring back the Czar? Maybe that *would be* their 'democratic will.' But it would **not** be in their best interests! Only workers who are forward-minded—who are the vanguard of their class—can really be counted on to perceive the class interests of the workers as a whole—and that means the Party! Starry-eyed dreaming is not materialist, nor is it dialectical. More, it's **counter-revolutionary**—plain and simple! We're trying to preserve the Revolution against *horrendous* odds, comrade! This is not the time to slacken in our resolve—nor is it time to allow bourgeois notions of 'rights' or petty-bourgeois, anarchist hogwash about 'autonomy' and 'spontaneity' frustrate what the forward-minded have a duty to do! Hard times call for hard measures—it's not pretty, comrade! It's not easy. But, we must trust that it is *necessary*—or the greatest hope of workers' emancipation since the Commune will be sacked and swept away on the dung heap of history! That's why theory is so important now. And that's why it's undisciplined, petty-bourgeois adventurism that pretends to come up with theory with no solid basis in reality—anarchism, ultra-leftism—hooliganism and banditry!—which is *the greatest enemy* of our work. If you wanna go to some liberal coffee-house and debate the finer points of modern art with your anarchist friends—that's fine, Theodor—get that outta your system, if you need to—but then—COME BACK HOME! And feel grateful that you don't have the pressing problems facing your very life and death everyday, like Comrade Lenin and Comrade Trotsky and all our Bolshevik brethren, allowing you to go to such artsy coffee-houses and get drunk on dreams of idealistic irresponsibility—while meanwhile, the rest of us are *working*—and working **hard**—to make a world where you can one day be free!!"

Theodor had nothing to say. Old Max was supported by the other comrades in the cell, and his blistering lambasting of Theo's call for freedom left him with a head unclear. Was Theo just a dilettante? Was he being influenced by petty-bourgeois notions? He thought to Katya, and all her friends. How many of them were workers like him? Not many, he had to admit. Some were from the upper classes, rebel children of the rich; most of the rest were not workers, but work-resisters, work-*avoiders*, priding themselves on avoiding wage-slavery by taking up a host of schemes, from digging in dustbins for food to procuring and selling black market items—from drugs to contraceptives to themselves—to various and sundry petty larcenies. Maybe they *did* represent alien class interests, as Max said, as Lenin had polemicized. Maybe they were not proletarian, but lumpen proletarian, or petty-bourgeois, or even the rulers of the world themselves, on a cheap holiday, a youthful diversion, before they'd return to the welcoming arms of their parents, and take their places among them.

Maybe, Katya . . .

But—**bullshit!** Opportunism came in many colours. And democracy was sacred, even if the people trying for it were nothing but "ignorant peasants"—or déclassé individualists who liked to think for themselves, who actually liked to enjoy themselves a little, and not wait till the Revolution. Democracy was essential to revolution, and whomever pointed it out, be they left or right or centrist, they had a point that could not be disputed. Opportunism was yellow, in the Second International; who knows?—was it too much of a stretch to see that opportunism could now be red?

Theodor left the meeting, wrestling with his party loyalty, his own instincts to fall in line and conform to it, and his biting need to question. Where was he going? Could he stand alone in such a Germany, where everything was opposing factions of political loyalty, fascists and communists and socialists and militarists and monarchists, and nobody in the world could do anything without the support of friends? He wasn't an anarchist. He did not buy the idea that society could resolve its problems with no organization whatsoever. In a world where capitalist armies still held sway, what would be the fate of a federation of autonomous collectives, even if that *were* the right way? It would be crushed by the forces of reaction. That was common sense. So, you needed some kind of government, some kind of structure, or the whole thing would fall, not only into chaos, but into sitting ducks just waiting, little commune by little commune, for the enemies to march upon them each in turn, and slaughter all hope.

Practicality. That's what Theodor wrestled with now. What could be done, really, actually, had to take precedence over what could be dreamed about. And, as a person who had grown up in the working class, mired in struggle and repression, he had a great attraction to hard-nosed pragmatists who, after all, had overthrown both Czar and Kerensky, both feudalism and capitalism, and repelled the armies of the Old Regime and the fourteen capitalist nations which marched beside them and sought the Communists' ruin. Maybe Max was right. Maybe this was not the time to point fingers of blame. After all, it was pretty easy to criticize something from the outside. How much harder it would be to be in the bloody arena, and question the efficacy of your fists, when that's all you had?

Yet, he couldn't let it go. The anarchists had a point, too. Kronstadt was sailors, some of the same sailors that had overthrown the Czar—and it was to defend their rights that they rose against the Bolshevik government. Theory! You could argue *anything*, it seemed, and dress it up with clever words! Dialectical logic became mere tricks of the pen and the mind if it made something that was tyranny into something which free people should defend. As much as he hated Germany, and scraping a living in lumpen proletarian ways, working precarious odd jobs and stealing potatoes and selling bits of leather he'd ripped from the overhead straps of trams to eat—

he'd much rather be here than in Russia now. And that was where it all resolved. He was sick of politics.

Katya was privileged. But was not Lenin privileged, too? People starved on the streets of Moscow. But Lenin and Trotsky did not starve. There were something like thirty-six different classes of rationing and housing imposed by the Bolsheviks now. (That was documented by many people who had been there lately, from famous people like Emma Goldman and Nestor Makhno and Voline, to personal acquaintances like that Swiss friend of Katya's, the closet bomb-maker, magnet-enthusiast and toilet-roll-poet Sebastien, to Theo's own close comrade and still-loyal Communist, Nadia.) And, necessity or not, those in power were being taken care of whilst their supposed comrades were eating human flesh to get by.

Theo could not accept what Max was saying. Even if his own head could not justify it, his heart was against Max. Dictatorship was dictatorship, and if it was, then dialectically speaking, the quantity of the Revolution had transformed it into its qualitative opposite. The thesis of proletariat had clashed with the antithesis of secretariat, synthesizing into this "Soviet Socialist Republic." A republic—not a democracy—no more democratic than any bourgeois republic—and from all reports, actually far, far less. Russia was not worth defending any more, if it wasn't a worker's democracy. No. It was a bureaucracy, and if it was workers in that bureaucracy, then they were workers no more. No matter that the people who agreed with him most were not workers, either. Truth was truth. And lies were lies, however prettily they were constructed and arranged. You could dress up tyranny anyway you liked. But it was ugly, no matter what "art" or "theory" was hung from its tentacles.

But where did all this leave Theo? Alone, alone. He walked the streets in a daze. He'd never felt more depressed, more disillusioned. His Papa was dying. He himself was starving. Germany was going mad. And, he thought, he might well soon go mad with it.

Never was he more attracted to Katya. Her politics were simpler than his, and also in their way, more practical. She had resolved her tendency's conflict between individual and collective. As a human being—not as some elite "vanguard" operative, but a plain and simple *human being*—no better and no worse than anybody else—she decided what she wanted to do, and she *did* it. If the fascists were bothering her, she fought them—fighting as dirty and unprincipled as they fought, outdoing them at their own game. If she needed something from the society, she *took* it—directly, with no justification, much less orders from on high. And she resolved her conflict between her individual sovereignty and the will of her collective by standing with her chosen community, her friends, her comrades, which were her family, choosing to stand with them of her own free volition. She happened to be surrounded by other individualists, and they decided together to act, as free men and women, whether beating up fascists, or stealing and scamming the big department stores, or finding the best, choicest delicacies tossed away in the rich people's dustbins in the West End, or producing art and literature and propaganda, or a hundred other things which struck them in the moment, gave them pleasure—and yet contributed to the same class war and sabotage of the state that Theodor had been fighting actively since he was fifteen with all his "seriousness."

Her friends agreed, mostly. Together, they acted in the best way that individuals can to advance their personal will and their personal pleasure: *collectively.* She called it "Mutual Aid," citing the anarchist Kropotkin's many works, including a posthumous work on *Ethics*, of which she'd somehow gotten some pages of the unfinished manuscript, passed along from friend to friend, comrade to comrade, beginning with some inspired anonymous Russian rebel who had supposedly smuggled it from Kropotkin's apartment hours after he'd died in the Soviet Union, before the Bolsheviks could steal and suppress it. (The authenticity of these pages was admittedly dubious. Perhaps, over the several sets of handwriting present on the oily, tea-stained pages, over its two-and-a-half-year journey through the frontiers between there and here, some anarchist equivalents of saints or spirit-mediums had channelled the late thinker, spirit-writing his words from the atheist afterlife. Sebastien's jest—though the documents were brought to the circle through his contacts, and taken seriously enough—whomever truly authored them.)

Katya wanted to quit Berlin, get a farm somewhere, and *live.* Form a little bubble of sense in the increasing insanity of the world. Where Theo had before condemned this as utopian, as irresponsible, as blind even, he now toyed with the idea of joining her. Maybe it *was* putting your head in the sand. But, if he was powerless over the forces of the world, unable to influence it, unable to change it, then what would be so wrong with just dropping out of it altogether?

Katya welcomed his feelings. She, too, had wrestled much with cynicism about the world, and her depression was like a cancer, eating away at her heart and soul, threatening to ruin her, to kill her. The great strikes of September, and the brief revolutionary stand of the workers in Saxony in October, had yielded nothing but repression, and the rising of Hitler's Nazis in Munich in November. Though Hitler was in jail, now, his movement was more alive than ever in the wake of the Munich "Beer Hall Putsch." Things seemed darker and darker by the month, by the week. It was harder and harder, now, to have hope.

The first task of a revolutionary is the same as the first task of any human being: to survive. And more and more, it seemed this world was no place to do that.

"We could really do it, you know," she smiled to him in her apartment, with a few young people sleeping off their drunks on the floors, herself in the bed beside a sleeping Guaril. Theo was coming to feel this commune-building the only practical alternative to despair, even if the commune was simply this apartment in the middle of war-mad Berlin. He felt better, lying a while on the great bed with her, his head on Guaril's chest, as she kissed him from his lightly-furred breast down his belly and middle to his thighs and calves and toes, kneeling finally at the foot of the bed and rubbing his feet.

"You really think so?" he said, bringing Guaril's sleepy arm round him and nestling there.

"Yes, liebling. I've an inheritance coming, from my great aunt, who's always loved me. She's in Switzerland now, convalescing from her sicknesses. But she won't last much longer, I'm sorry to say. She's been writing me letters over the past year, though lately her health's been too bad even to write. She hates my family—my mother, my father, my brothers. She's leaving everything of hers to me—nearly a hundred million marks—that's *pre-war value*, liebling—what it used to buy, in *gold*. Of course, all those millions of marks wouldn't buy us a couple of eggs now, but my great auntie was smart enough to know that the old Fatherland was gonna lose the War, so she invested in gold, and stuck it all in some Swiss bank vault. It's equivalent to trillions and trillions, now. It'll get us that farm in Bavaria—*and* to spare. I say we travel for a while, and look round, y'know? Somewhere where we could all live."

Obligations. This was the sad song of Theodor. He couldn't leave now, as much as he wanted to. He could not leave his Papa.

"Bring 'im along!" she exhorted. "Sure, Theo! He's welcome in my universe—sweet old man! Let him live his last days outside this decaying, polluted ruin of a city."

"He'll never come."

"Why not?"

"Because, Katya, he's—he's a lot like me. He sticks it out where he is. He doesn't just leave. Even if he should."

Katya nodded sadly. Very well, she said. She would stay around, until the inevitable overtook Theo's Papa. And then? Then, she'd leave, and take her little tribe with her. She asked Theo, again, to come.

Theo nodded.

"I think I very well might," he said, almost as a promise to her. But then, he had to get back home. His Papa was sick, and needed him.

Guaril awoke later, and listened to Katya's telling him of the wrangling Theo had been involved in with his comrades, down at the newly-rented Spartakist headquarters. Guaril was sympathetic. Theory was good, he affirmed; but, anything could be constructed, any ontology, if one accepted certain axiomatic premises. If you thought that Russia now was the hope of workers' revolution, then all of it followed. You had to be a partisan, a soldier. That was not where Theo was, Guaril realized, Katya affirmed. Theo was a worker, first and foremost. And, as a worker, he could not stomach lies, nor privilege. Had he not broken away from the Social Democracy of his youth and family tradition, because of this very same bureaucracy that was ruining the workers' movement? Bureaucrats were nothing new. They'd been weighing down workers' politics here in Germany for at least two generations, their treacheries shown in the many sell-outs of the Second International back in the nineteenth century and down to their support of the Great War, and just now the sell-out of the German Revolution in Saxony, when the Zentrale of the Third International decided to abandon their support of the Saxon workers in a closed-door meeting at Chenmitz—or so the rumours said. Every country in the world with a workers' movement had similar stories of bureaucratic betrayal, Theodor knew. It seemed in this epoch, the bureaucracy was rising as a class, just as the bourgeoisie had risen from the ruins of feudalism, a middling layer within the feudal power structure. The bureaucrats were the new middling layer. And they, as their predecessors before them, were co-opting the movements of the poor, to install themselves into power on their backs.

This was the "theory" that Theo came to in those months, that winter and early spring in Berlin as 1923 passed like an understated whirlwind into 1924, wrestling with problems of socialism, anarchy, and the fate of humanity. Katya and Guaril and even the sceptic Johanna contributed to the discussion, and there were many friends of Katya who lent their minds to the formulation of the differences Theo had with Bolshevism. Sebastien met Nadia at Katya's pad over those long days and nights of debate, the latter the only Party-member who dared contribute to the project besides Theo himself—though the Polish comrade thought of Red Rosa, and her bravery in defying the status quo of Eduard Bernstein's reformism a generation ago, despite being a Pole and a Jew and a woman not yet twenty-five in what was then (and was still) a German, gentile, old boy's world. Nadia thought to emulate the example of their martyr, even if she couldn't do it openly. Sebastien, ever anarchist, of the more "individualist" tendency, had some quite spirited debates with the staid and loyalist Nadia, who more than held her own. Very soon, both of them had moved rather quietly toward each other, declaring themselves "autonomists" (somewhere between communists and anarchists, they told their closest friends); and, just as quietly, and just as quickly, Nadia and Sebastien moved towards one another relationally, the two never seen apart by the first weeks of April. They were the first to leave Berlin and Katya's scene, though whether the new couple headed east or west was anyone's guess.

The theories the little circle came up with were published in renegade leftist publications in the first months of 1924, most notably *Die Aktion,* whose once-art-critic publisher, Franz Pfemfert, was an acquaintance of Katya's from the old Dada days in Zurich. But then they collected all their thoughts into one extended pamphlet which they began to distribute on May 1st of 1924 at the Mayday Parade, where they gave away nearly a thousand of them. Their words won them no friends; but they had each other. They all came to a closer friendship over those months, these young anarchists and artists and bohemians and bums in the salon of Katya and her comrades. People spoke of the "new class" in Russia. They spoke of Rosa Luxemburg's *Marxism or Leninism?*, a pamphlet that was hard to get now, but spoke volumes, written shortly before Red Rosa's martyrdom at the hands of Noske's Frei Korps whilst still in prison for sedition, prophesying the coming doom of workers' politics at the hands of the Bolsheviks. The anarchists were less into theory than the communists, at least economic, "class theory." Yet, the communists seemed almost drunk with their theory, making of it less honest investigations into the social problem than a series of dogmas and doctrines. Somewhere between them, this was where Theo, Katya, Guaril, and the rest sought their solutions, and debate was heated and richly textured in the taverns and cafés and late-night rent parties in the flats and town-homes of their scene. What to do about it? This was the telling question. But, before they could get to the future, there was a need for analysis of the present. And this is what Theo did, along with his comrades, in between scrambling for the next mark, the next meal.

Theo's Papa was sick, and as the spring waned to summer, the sickness became more and more acute and debilitating. Theo told him to go to a sanatorium, to go to Switzerland, perhaps, and recover. But the old man just laughed.

"Even if we had the cash, Theodor," he said, slumped in his broken chair in the kitchen, with one of his many pilsners before him, which he drank against the urgent reprimands of his doctors, "there's no 'recovering' for me. You know that, and I know that. This old worker is going to his final reward—death, and dust, Theodor. I'll proudly spit in Jesus *and* the Devil's eye—and fade into nothingness. I'm a socialist to the end, my son . . ."

Theo loved his father. During those months, their conversations grew more and more serious, more and more profound. Ricard Priser wanted no bullshit now. He spoke openly of his failed marriage, of the sadness he had considering his daughter, a proud, "New Woman" with money and a career in the thriving film industry—who, rumours said, was considering the National Socialist Party. The mother was a devout Catholic, now, which, to Ricard, was just as bad. He believed in his politics like his religion. It gave him comfort in his last hours, along with his beer and his friends, whom he still saw, they coming over to share their sadness and their awkward jokes at the side of the dying man. Theo came closer than he'd ever been to really *getting* his old man, and having the old man get him. They spoke of Theodor's recent issues with his party, with communism generally, and while not agreeing with his even more leftist vision, Ricard Priser found some sense in his son's new revelations.

For there is something in being a worker that distrusts hierarchy, that distrusts the intellectual. Papa Priser often thought his son mixed up with something elitist, and radical in all the wrong ways. Murderers, he thought the Bolsheviks, men with no principles beyond that of *Realpolitik.* The ends justifying the means. That's no way to run a government, he'd grumbled often to his son, and he was encouraged that Theodor was no longer an automaton of the Party. Ricard wanted peace. But, he knew well that peace would not come now. Things were just too crazy now. And he knew they'd likely get crazier.

"I'm glad I'm dying," he said to Theo one night in latest June.

"Why, Papa?"

"Because I know this world's gonna get really ugly in the next years. I worry about ya, son. But I know you can't do something you don't believe in."

"No. I never could."

"Right. I know. . . . What I mean to say to ya, son, is that I respect you, for the fight you've made. I'm no friend of the bourgeoisie; I'm no friend of the bureaucrats, either. I stay with the Social Democracy out of loyalty to what they once were. But, I know. I *know.* I know they won't be the solution in the future."

"No, Papa. I don't think they will."

"And those Spartakists won't either."

"I agree."

"So. What *is* the solution?"

Before Theo could come up with some kind of answer, the father had gone on, chuckling a wry and defeated chuckle.

"The Nazis," he said, in the tone of prophesy. "They're the solution, son. They're where this thing is headed. People are easily led. Fuck! *I* was easily led—all these years. Your big sister's got the right idea. Get in good with those fuckers, and your life'll be good in the future."

"God, Papa! I can't do that!"

"I know, son. And I love ya for that more than you can know. The Jewish people are the *chosen* people. Never doubt that, son. It's their unhappy fate to be the sacrificial lamb, the scapegoat, that will be sacrificed to make this Deutschland proud of herself again. Pride is so important, my son. And those bastard Allies after the War, they blamed *us* for it. That was their mistake. Because Deutschland *is* gonna rise again—make no mistake—and it's gonna rise up with some madman pushing hate at its head. And then? . . . Then, son, the whole world's gonna *end* . . ."

Theo's father knew his prophesy for his nation and his class was grim and apocalyptic. He knew that the world in the future would be horrible, beyond the dreams of any dark modern artist he never understood. Gothic and terrible. The return of the Devil himself into the world. Madness. That was the fate he saw. And he did not envy his son his health. Ricard wanted to die.

Theo wept. He loved his father—so much! He hugged him, kissed his cheek, his neck. The father, drunkenly, wept also. But he kept himself afloat. He was among the privileged. He would not have to see Germany, and the world, in ruins.

Theo listened as his father told him he wanted to die at home, here, in this little hovel, which was his place in the world, for better or worse. But it wasn't fated to be. He collapsed one night in July, and Theodor ran down the street to a payphone and called an ambulance. Theodor's father was brought to the city hospital, a big, open floor with many beds in it, cavernous, echoey, anything but privacy under those vaulted ceilings. Here, his father would die.

Theodor contacted his mother and sister, who came near the dawn. They'd been living on the West End, in better circumstances since they'd ditched the old man, and made for themselves something of a fortune. The mother was a wasted woman, dark and morose, dressed in black and a veiled bonnet, wearing a big silver crucifix and praying a rosary. Theodor's big sister was a businesswoman, strong and self-sufficient in her smart suit-jacket dress. She was a modern woman, Theo thought, much like his Katya. But, of course, "modern" told you next to nothing. She was blonde and striking, taller than Theodor by nearly a head. Her icy, Aryan blue eyes accused him in the dawn, as her sharp, clipped, rapid words soon did, telling him that he should have called sooner, that he was remiss.

"I'm sorry," he said.

"Well," she said, "I suppose it's useless now. Mother's very distraught."

Theodor wondered at this. After all his pain, staying with his Papa, nursing him through the agonies of his cancer these last long years, it seemed a little remiss to be pointing the finger now.

After all, where had *she* been?

"Yeah," Theodor said. "Let's go see him, eh?"

"Right. Let's go."

The two siblings walked through the graveyard of terminal beds, her high heels and his work boots echoing on the dirty linoleum of the hospital floor amidst the chatters of a hundred dying souls, to find the bed where their father lay, as if in state. They found him awake.

"Hey, Vati!" the sister smiled to him, as if she'd just left him yesterday, though it had been fully three years since they'd last spoken.

The old man was beginning to be delirious. He saw his daughter as some woodland sprite in his fantasy, half taken from bedtime stories told to him by his own mother, when she was around, which was a rarity, half taken from Wagner, whom the elder Priser felt was the most wonderful composer the world had ever known. Yes. A woodland sprite. And there, beside her, a pixie. Freya, he mumbled, and beside her, Frey.

"Hey, Papa," Theodor said, as he'd said over and over for the last years.

"I am grateful," the old man pronounced. "Grateful. I have St. Joseph's death. A happy death. With my loved ones all around me."

The highfalutin tenor of the old man's language did not abate that morning. All he could do was sing the praises of saints and gods, forgetting forty years of atheism and defiance, and link them with his surroundings. It was for both Theodor and his sister rather uncomfortable. There would be no bedside reunions of any sense there that morn.

Theodor's mother came at last to his father's side. She kissed him, and placed medals of her favourite saints on his chest, medals from Lourdes and Fatima and a dozen other places where Mary had supposedly appeared. She whispered in an attempt to comfort that these medals, already holy, had been made holier by the blessings of bishops and cardinals in every locale they'd come from. The father accepted this, not seeming too aware, and still talking in poetry when he talked at all.

And then, he died.

That was all. It was sudden, though it was evident that the process of his death had been proceeding for years, years and years, and Theodor's mother and sister were alike unaware of the tragedy that he saw: they'd been absent the whole time.

They went out for an early luncheon, the sister paying, a little place, quite nice, actually, on one of the main boulevards of Berlin. Mother cried, mother mourned. She felt she was to blame, somehow, crippled by her Catholicism, her unnatural guilt. Sister had none of this. She spoke very matter-of-fact, very coldly and clearly. Things happened. And the father, after all, had been no saint.

"No," Theodor admitted.

"He had no head for this world," the sister continued. "He had no sense of discipline. That's why Mother had to leave him. He spent money like a madman! What did he think? That he was some kinda bourgeois, with a license to spend like that? I'm sorry Theodor, Mother. But it's times like this when you must face facts. I'm sorry. I don't want to say bad things right now. But he—he was the reason I had to do without. That Mother had to do without. That you, Theodor, had to do without."

"I've got no complaints, sis," Theo said, cold and impersonal. He did not like his sister. And he knew she didn't much care for him. Let her go on ad nauseum about the old man; that was her right. But, damned if *he*, Theo, would contribute to the sacrilege.

"Well, that's fine," she said dismissively. "I don't mean to speak ill of the dead. . . . I suppose we'll cremate him."

"That's what he wanted. He wants his ashes scattered over the river."

"Yes, that's fine. Save us some cash, I bet. That's one thing he *did* do for us, I suppose . . ."

Theodor had not seen his sister in three years, and before that it had been longer. She was senior to him by but two and a half years, but they seemed long years. She was beyond him, beyond his class. She had that upward mobility drive Marxists don't acknowledge as important. She would make a name for herself. She knew better than to dabble in politics with the communist she figured her brother was. She hated that, all that. The workers were deficient, she thought, or they wouldn't be workers. This Deutschland, as all capitalist countries, was a treasure trove, if only you had the ambition and the brains to claim its wealth. Sure, the crisis; sure, the treaty. But even in the crisis, the intelligent could find opportunities, if they only were clear-headed, hard-working, and had vision. Even the deterioration of the Mark could be used to the advantage of the smart and resourceful. She explained that the film company she was rising up the rungs of right now had found a clever way to exploit the situation, borrowing in Papiermarks for its projects, then paying back the investors a few months later in money that had decreased significantly in value since they'd gotten the loans—maximizing their profits handsomely with each production! That's why the film industry here in Germany was thriving now, hundreds of companies making films all over, many tens in Berlin alone. Faced with the lack of cash to make the dazzling sets of our Hollywood competitors, we Germans have created a whole new way to make film, she said with pride—the "Expressionist" style, making the most of poor sets by designing them purposefully unreal, *surreal*, the perfect complement to the superior, intellectual themes they tackled, creating a genre of film making Theodor's sister was certain would influence world cinema for generations to come. The Fatherland would be whole again, she intoned with sharp and certain confidence. That would mean making the best of an unjust situation, imposed on the country by foreigners and their collaborationist allies right here at home. That would mean ridding the country of all the communists and Jews that were ruining it, and delivering the common people to their doom.

Theodor breathed hard. While she didn't mean to dabble in "politics," her nasty anti-Semitism and hatred of the class she'd been born into was coming out, despite her honest efforts not to go there. Theodor casually mentioned that his new lover was a Jewess, and her family was one of the leading shipping magnates in this part of Germany. But she hated her family as much as she hated the fucking Nazis.

"We can all learn a lot," Theo said grandly, "from her example."

"Yes, I suppose," the sister dismissed. She knew her brother was bound for no good; his dating one of *them* just solidified the thought. She sighed, and ate the rest of her meal, as did Theo and his mother, in silence. Then, it was time to go.

They cremated the old man, and scattered his ashes over the Spree, as was his final wishes. None of them understood it, really, what made it important, the river, the ashes. But, as Sister said, it saved them a bundle, forgoing a funeral and a burial and all that. Sister then disappeared, Mother in tow.

Theo never saw them again.

Chapter 9

Summer was grand, despite all the pain. The threesome of Katya, Theo, and Guaril continued to grow and flower, despite the ugliness of Berlin and the world. For, there was Beauty still.

The Tiergarten was a glorious stretch of nature within the city. Katya, Theo, and Guaril all wondered aloud at the wonder of civic planning and civic art, that even in the midst of all the ugliness of government, all its horrendous and useless fixations, war, repression, the building of prisons and tenements and sewers that did not work, there could still be something of Beauty in its undertakings. Perhaps this was the hand of God, Theo surmised, in defiance of his Spartakist training and Social Democratic upbringing; perhaps it was a happy accident, Katya though aloud, the kind of thing that was random in history, the kind of thing she suspected was at the heart of everything, despite the mechanistic and deterministic understandings of her time; but perhaps it was just something to enjoy, and not to question, Guaril said, as was the brilliant August sunlight, gentle and lemon yellow, blending the colours of the leaves and the tree bark and the grass and the flowers into the pastel pallor of an Impressionist painting. So entranced were they, with the wonder and beauty of their surroundings, and even, they dared imagine, their times, that they barely noticed the Brownshirts marching down the path, halting them with—"Whadya doin' here, Gypsyboy?!"

"What's that?" Guaril said.

"You," they said, almost in one voice—"You're not allowed here, boy. Get your black ass outta our park—or there'll be trouble!"

Guaril was in the mood to fight; they all were. But there were ten stormtroopers to their three, and everyone knew—both groups—that the SA could do pretty much what they wanted in the city now. Cursing them, they left the park, deciding on a whim to go down to the constabulary, to formally protest the toughs as the unruly bastards they were. Katya saw no point in it, but a feeling lingered Theo that such things as "law" and "a case" might still matter, that a record of the SA's harassment might help someone someday. Guaril went along with it, curious, suspending his judgement. But the cop at the station told them that those "fine young men" had just done what they had done out of civic duty. In fact, just a few years ago, the city of Dusseldorf passed an ordinance banning all Roma from the public parks—not just camping caravans, but *all of them*. Though the same law had not yet been enacted in Berlin, the cop told them he thought it a fine idea, and assured them that such a law would soon be in effect. If the "good old boys of Deutschland" wanted to prohibit social scum from polluting their parks, he would offer no resistance—and would damn well encourage it, if any of the boys had been his own sons.

Shocked, angry, but not really surprised, the three left the station, and trekked back to their home, which was Katya's. The two men had moved in more or less permanently, Theo unable to make the rent since his father's death, Guaril having been kicked out of his flat without notice or reason earlier in the month. They spoke a while, angry words, and words consoling, but ultimately fruitless. In the pregnant pause that followed, they decided to make love.

Guaril knelt before Katya, his face soon immersed in her sex, deliciously tasting her wet, swelling essences, Theo behind him, driving his manhood into the supple, sinuous curves of his daddy's backside. They played blissfully in the garden of one another, Guaril entering Katya, entering Theo, kissing and tasting, Theo playing boy and girl and souls intermediate, Katya welcoming them into herself and then thrusting into them with sex toys of wood and metal and carved ginger—fingers, tongue, and toes in turn. It was beautiful, the moments they shared as the golden afternoon waned to twilight, such that, afterwards, all they wanted to do was sleep in each other's arms.

They slept, spooning each other, on pillows strewn with white rose petals. They'd soaked them in a chloral hydrate-ether elixir, then bitten into them and tasted them on each other's lips till they'd drifted into dreaming, Guaril on one side, his strong arm flexed even in sleep, Theo cradled warmly on the other, Katya in the middle, engulfed and engulfing. The canopy bed was grand, a relic of Katharina the daughter of bourgeois privilege—one of the few things she'd brought with her into the flat from the mansions of her childhood. Most of her furniture had been found in the trash, accounting for its age and worn-out condition, as well as its lack of any matching scheme. The few nicer things had been pinched by friends from the lobbies of hotels—the oriental divan in the further room, for instance, its vermilion upholstery amongst the only furniture skins here that did not seem leprous. But Katharina, as her mother still called her, had great pride in having acquired the stuff without having had to pay anything for it. It was part of her philosophy, of salvaging the world's refuse, of living—*and living well*—in the shadows of a decaying society.

"My mother told me once," she said to her lovers later, in the light of the full moon, coming in through wispy, silvery clouds through the dirty glass of the windows, "or, rather, she asked me— 'why don't you buy yourself some proper furniture, Katharina, that would match, that would have some style?' I told her I preferred what I had. She told me, a little smugly, but mostly in real puzzlement, that she would become very, very depressed indeed, if she had to get her furniture out of the trash. I told her, I myself would find it very, very depressing to have had to spend money for it."

Katya smiled in the night.

"She told me, 'I suppose that's the difference between you and me.' And I told her she was right."

Guaril and Theo loved her, each in his own way, truly and unjealously. They had no sense of ownership, both believing as strongly as she did in non-monogamy. This was simply the right way to live, to love. It didn't matter that the lifestyle hadn't been thought up much before now, as far as they knew, that it was a function of what they all recognized as a decadent Berlin society. They were decadent, too; but they revelled in their decadence. Decadence was the mother of freedom.

And, besides, what was "wrong" with it? Even as they embraced decadence, they felt a moral superiority to the dead values of Christianity and bourgeois society. Marriage, one-to-one existence, even if it could be rescued from its patriarchal and propertarian trappings, was simply a lacklustre way to live. There was so much more to being three than two, just as two was more than being one.

Yet, they theorized, three was more, too, than four or five. They knew each other, intimately, and were content within their sacred triad, in which each was loved by two good friends instead of one; yet there was still a sense of something private among them, something very hard to appreciate unless you were there within the loving trinity. Guaril wondered, though, at Friedrich Engels' *Origin of the Family*, and the idea of the group marriages of the era before civilisation, and the possibility of expanding their ménage to include still others in their love. Each of them wondered to their commune, and the family they might have there. Consanguine, or almost; confraternal surely. All friends, all lovers—what was the difference, after all? Love for most people was a fleeting thing, in divorce, separation, death, or in the living death of being "stuck" with one another. Love, for the fortunate souls of this ménage, could be an ongoing thing, as one person moved from another to another, only to return. A whole philosophy spawned among them, though they wrote none of it down. So much better to *live* it!

And Johanna. She came to visit, of an evening or dawn twilight, to get her sense back after working her trade. She took the pleasures of Katya, and teased Theo and Guaril, not unkindly, with fantasies she half meant to fulfil. Surely, sometime, of a midnight revel, she would draw both men into her arms, and punish them for the masculinity she hated, which they represented to her despite their feminine sides. She hated men. She hated them sexually; and, too, as an *idea.* She spoke of parthenogenesis, and a book she liked called *Herland*, an American feminist fantasy book of the last decade by the American Charlotte Perkins Gilman she'd read in English, which chronicled a lost civilisation of women, high up in the Andes in South America, which had lived for centuries without even *seeing* a man. She spoke, too, of what she called "the elder civilisations," the oldest civilisations: the social insects, ants and wasps and bees, most all of whom were sisterhoods, with just a few male drones to impregnate the queen, and then to be stung to death and discarded at the end of every season. These civilisations, she would smile with goddess-like confidence, had been living in their cities since before the dinosaurs walked the earth, hundreds of millions of years ago. They'd be there when Man and His history and His patriarchal, genocidal tribalism ("nationalism," they called it now) had wiped Himself from the face of the earth.

But, she liked Theo and Guaril, not least of all because they so liked each other. She felt the only men to keep around after her own radical feminist revolution would be the queer ones, who could help along the project of reproduction if her parthenogenesis schemes should prove too difficult. Drones, she smiled, like in a beehive. You'd only need a few, in a society of millions of beautiful women. And, she smiled, embracing them, Theo and Guaril should be among that elite. She wouldn't, she cackled sharply, even advocate stinging them to death once their sperm dried up in their little enlarged clits.

All this was, of course, out of step with most people around them, even many of the anarchists and bohemians who frequented their slum salon. But, among the rest, there were just as many ideas, just as apparently crazy and out of step, and people came to a consensus that consensus was not the best thing. Live, and let live, was the least of their mottoes. In the highest sense, it was possible to actually *dig* (as the hep jazzmen would say) the alternatives of lifestyle and philosophy that grew in their little community, among their little subsets and cliques. Everyone was together, precisely in their apartness. After all, this Berlin in the Weimar 'twenties was nothing if it not eclectic, and daring, a vanguard of sorts for all the rest of the world. Whilst their small circle explored their sexual and spiritual and political paths to enlightenment, there were countless other circles in and round Berlin that were doing the same, as evidenced by the journals that proliferated. *Die Freundschaft* and *Der Eigenen, Die Freundin* and *Der Insel,* and thirty other publications explored queer and alternative sexuality. *Der Sturm* and *Die Aktion* stood out amongst all the other magazines that spoke of radical art and radical politics, and how they intersected. And then magazines like *Der Strom* and *Blatter fur Menschenrecht* did a fine job of straddling the divide between radical sexuality and radical politics. All these organs were as flags fluttering proudly red and proudly black over the crumbling towers of Old Deutschland—brazen standards of the revolution shaking those towers' foundations. This was another positive spin on the term "decadence." After all, what was "decaying" all around them, if not the evil of evils—*civilisation itself?*

Of course, there were plenty of people outside their circles. And these were intent on exploiting or, conversely, eradicating this decadence. After their failed "beer hall putsch" last November had landed a lot of those ugly Nazi bastards in jail, some of the hopeful in the centre and the left had prophesied the death of their movement. But the defeat of their rebellion and the jailing of their leaders hadn't deterred the rest of them in the least. If anything, it seemed to give them renewed strength, making them seem heroic and genuinely rebellious in the eyes of the undecided, giving them a host of martyrs to confirm the myth of persecution which they'd been selling for years: the good, Aryan German people, held hostage by the Bolshevist, liberal, leftist, Jewish conspiracy that had taken their government from them and sold them to the foreigners. The SA continued to grow, their ranks swelling with pimps and professors. They continued to harass people on the street, fighting bitter battles with Communists and Socialists and just passers-by, generally winning people over to thoughts of some grand and glorious past era.   And they were working on the younger generation, too, their "Hitler Youth" a kind of boy scouts for National Socialism, with thousands of young boys joining every week since their founding two years ago—even if many of the boys were attracted to the camping and the bicycling as much as the uniforms and the marching and the propaganda. The hope of the Nazis was surely to train young kids to fill future Brownshirt uniforms when they got a little taller. On the other, more adult side of things, Nazi sympathizers were publishing numerous diatribes, fighting the ideological battle to compliment the street fights, intellectuals all over society writing books and giving lectures and making films "proving" the science of racism, pushing for eugenics, selling the idea of purity and strength—as if such things came not from choice and life, but from blood and genes.

What they were talking about was, of course, nonsense. But somehow, appeals to some mythic past were more salient to a regressive society than the Leftists' vision of some mythic future. It was winning out. Societies in decay long for some past time, just as hopeful, developing societies long for the future.   The latter is restless, frustrated with things as they are, whilst the former is fearful, longing for a lost stability. Weimar was many things—risky, eclectic, cultured, experimental—but fearless it was not.   Its government was a coalition of moderate parties who were just holding back the flood. And everyone had a feeling it was a flood that would one day break the dam, drowning them all . . .

Katya was plagued more and more viciously by melancholia as the spring waned and the summer blazed past and the nights began again to grow longer. Her analysts proved, one after another, to be ineffective and unsympathetic. They talked nonsense, and went nowhere. And meanwhile, Katya slid further and further away. There were times she couldn't even get out of bed, for days and nights she'd lay there, barely eating, the heavy, stained purple curtains always drawn. Guaril and Theo tried to help, Theo massaging her, making sure she got some nourishment each day, Guaril singing her lullabies and laments he could still remember from his mother and grandmother, before he was taken away from their caravan by the government of Spain, many years ago. But the boys, too, felt more than a little affected by the ennui of Berlin.   Guaril found himself being followed, by Nazis, by Bullen, he wasn't sure. And Theo began to despair at the politics he'd been a partisan of just months before, at the very prospect of workers' emancipation. There were *two* classes the workers had to fight against now, and the direction of the movement seemed damned not to free itself, but to reckon the hegemony of one or another of these two rival, parasite oligarchies.

What would Germany look like if the Nazis won? Would it really be that different from a Germany where the Communists won? Different people would go to the camps, surely; but there'd be camps in either case. And the end of capitalism would lead not to socialism, not to anarchy, but to a new kind of social order, which owed nothing to the past, and would, more even than the rule of the bourgeoisie, sabotage and betray the future. The bureaucrats, be they organized under the party patronage machine of the Bolsheviks or the Nazis, would be even more against the workers, if such a thing were possible, than the bourgeoisie had been—precisely because they'd studied the workers so well in the course of their rising.

This was the meat of the pamphlets the salon began to write in earnest towards the middle and end of 1924, which Theo researched in the city libraries for hours and hours each day, pouring through statistics in journals and ledgers and the newest publications on economics. The Italian economy under Mussolini; the Russian economy under the New Economic Policy, and the War Communism of before; the economies of France, England, and the U.S.A. before and after the War; and the German economy as it moved from recession to depression and deeper still into abyss . . . Such things Theo studied, shared, and wrote about in tandem with his friends. They printed the pamphlets with Katya's money, and Guaril's cover art, and help from old friends like Nadia and Sebastien, who began by the fall to correspond from an address just outside Ascona, Switzerland. The pamphlets were distributed round town by the comrades among the salon, and their influence extended far beyond it.

And when there was objection to them, it wasn't just Brownshirts or bourgeois who levelled it.

Old Max got wind of it all. He called Theodor one night in October, at Katya's flat. How he got the number was a mystery; but he seemed to know an awful lot about how Theodor lived.

"Comrade," came the old, wizened voice across the phone-line, not angry, friendly rather, "we need to talk."

"Max?" Theodor said, incredulously. "How did you get this number?"

"Come, come," laughed the voice. "We've got a government, Theodor, who helps us. We've got an infrastructure. Whatta you got?"

"Max, I suppose you wanna know something about the pamphlets me and my friends've been writing."

"Sure, comrade, sure. That's kinda why I called ya. Ya ain't been to the meetings in a while. I suppose you know your dues ain't been paid in a while, either."

"Yeah, I know that. Of course I know that. I, er—I ain't had the money."

"Yeah, yeah, times are hard for all of us. *C'est la guerre, nicht wahr?* On the Seine and the Spree. On the Volga, too. You get a job yet?"

"Naw. Still lookin'."

"Yeah, yeah, times are hard for all of us. . . . I think I might be able to help ya."

"Really?"

Theo's voice was guarded. He was more than a little suspicious of his old friend, after all that had passed in the last year. He hadn't been to a cell meeting in months. Max's tirade against him still echoed illy in his heart and mind, even though it had been almost a year since they'd had the fight. He'd begun to be a little paranoid of Max, the Communists, and all but a few of his old comrades, truth be told. But, too, he was fairly desperate. He was inclined to listen.

"Yeah, comrade. I think I might be able to help ya. What say ya come down to the docks sometime, and we can talk?"

"Whereabouts?"

"Near the old warehouse. I still work there, ya know. Some of the fellas still do. We've held out. Even though a lotta the old SPD blockheads have joined up with the Nazis."

"Jesus!"

"Naw, comrade. Old Jesus has very little to do with it. It's a sign o' the times. There'll be a time in this country where there'll be just two ways to go: their way, or our way. . . . I know you kinda think I'm right, there, eh?"

Theo breathed.

"Yeah," he said. "I kinda do."

The smile over the line was almost audible.

"Good, comrade. Good. You might not be such an adventurer after all, eh?"

Theodor laughed despite himself. Old Max laughed along with him.

"C'mon down, brother," he said. "I think I've got a job for ya. All we need to do is talk a little business, first."

"Okay, Max. When?"

"How 'bout right now? Sure. I'm outta work in an hour. There's a place we Spartakists are meetin', a place near the warehouse. It's rough, but then, which one of us are millionaires?"

"I know I ain't."

"I know you ain't, brother. That's why we're talkin' . . ."

When Theo got off the phone, Katya was asleep, having slept most of the day. Guaril was chatting about Dada with a young, delicately-featured anarchist of intermediate or inverted gender, who had worn a feminine cast in *ihre Kleidung und ihre Merkmale,* in ihre clothing and features, but with unshaven legs and a soft furry stubble sie refused to pluck, like modest muttonchops round *ihre Ohren.* Sie had of late been using male pronouns to describe a consciously androgynous style, and then back to feminine ones again. Just last week, the pretty, handsome person had settled on the sometimes gender-neutral pronoun "sie"—though, who knows? Even this might be not enough to contain the person's potentials in the future. Sie had been one of the students who'd inspired others to compose group poetry on rolls of toilet paper, series of which by now formed a poem the size and quality of Joyce's *Ulysses,* a book sie had been devouring since it appeared in the radical bookseller's a few months ago. The toilet paper poetry had found many uses, and had had many contributors. Sie had composed at least a full roll with Erika, the motley-clad Romani woman with the German name. Erika's little baby Chevali, who was walking and talking now, had begun to contribute to the poetry, too—the child's nonsense sounds as cherished as the highly original groupings of "proper" words she'd been putting together of late, the ones she'd been talking to herself with in a long, unbroken dialogue—a crazy, advanced, elfin child Chevali was. The androgynous, once-womanly lesbian Teddi had contributed reams to the project, in between organizing all-night cruises for queers of all sexes and stripes down Berlin's rivers and canals out of the Domino Club, which the once-garçonne-now-sharper owned now with her/his partner, Gert. Robyn (or, Rob), the Irish Tinker folk singer, whose balding, gnomish head always sported a beaten fedora and whose skeletal arms cradled always a Ukrainian violin, had scratched many verses onto the rolls in drunken flights of midnight fancy, delighting in how the rips under his fountain pen complimented the violence of his imagery. Erik Boom!, the clown and contortionist and saboteur, had taken "volumes" of the poetry up with him whilst suspended above the Spree—wrapping the volumes (rolls) round him amidst his shackles like gauze round a mummy—and he'd managed to escape his bonds and straitjackets without disturbing the tensile integrity of a single stanza—all of which would be read before, during, and after the escapes. Al, the Yank banjo player from Chicago, who broke bottles of Clicquot Club ginger ale mingled with bootleg whiskey and bootleg gin over his war-wound iron kneecap when he'd had enough, and then would tear into blues and jazz and hill-billy improvisations on his sturdy, ragged instrument that would put Harry Reser to shame—scrawled nonsense verses onto the rolls during all-night jam sessions at the many rent parties they all threw, sometimes with his hands and sometimes with his feet— "photographic negatives" of his crazy, half-remembered lyrics in blobby, inky scribbles, backwards and upside down on the other side of the ponderous scrolls. Dozens of others had made their mark, all great geniuses in their way, and all but unknown. The originator selbst thought of two main purposes for the "post-Dada" poetry: the first being toilet paper—"You know—to give us something to read in the loo"—or to be sold to bourgeois art dealers who dealt with "edgy" things, making Duchamp's urinal into something people literally paid small fortunes for now, as the collectors passed it around between them in their endless dance of possession and control. The young artist's name had changed several times over the last two years, as sie had changed *ihre Studiums* at university from art to art history to art theory to art criticism before finally giving up on learning anything real about art from such stuffy, bourgeois institutions, and finally dropped out. *Ihren Namen*, lately, was "Siegfried," the name shifting with ihre shifting from feminine to masculine from Sieglinde, to Sigilind, to Sigi, to Sigmund over the last years. Siegfried had once identified as a "Tadpole," taking the mostly-pejorative lesbian subcultural term as a positive archetype, something deliberately undesirable, *proudly* ugly, as if to declare independence from the whole sordid dance of attraction; though now, that term, like every other bandied about in the queer, inverted world of Weimar Berlin, seemed hardly adequate for the unique soul who once used it for selbst. Few outside the circles of Katya's slum salon could understand the gender-rebel-artist that sie was. Judged as a woman—or at least, as something other than a man—sie had found selbst cut out of the line-up for the Dada exhibition called the *Dada-Messe* in 1920, where few besides Hannah Höch had been able to break through the man-dominated roster. Siegfried (who was a friend of Hannah's, as well as others of that scene, all the invisible non-male Dadaists of a history that would never be written), had given away many pieces of art over *ihre Jahre,* ihre years; the collage of Otto Gebuhr as Frederick the Great, mingling with faggots and dykes and queerer folk, all in the dirty, lovely acts of making love, was *ihrer Entstehung,* ihrer creation. And sie could care less that, other than the folks who passed this way, through the raging rent parties and the quiet, hungover afternoons of this flat, none would ever see ihre work, *ihre Künstlerishe Arbeit. Fuck history,* sie said often, yawning and laughing. *It's all just toilet-paper, in the end . . .*

Siegfried and Guaril had been laughing and flirting over the long afternoon and into the evening, postulating that the best and most unique art, like the best and most unique people, were never remembered, and that history, like property, was theft. But they'd fallen silent as Theo concluded his chat with Max.

Theo got his things together, and prepared to go.

"Where to, brother?" Guaril said, eyeing his jacket and his hat.

"Down to the docks," Theo answered, almost as if it were a question. "That was Old Max on the phone."

"Max? The commie?"

"Yeah."

"How'd he get our number?"

"I dunno. I don't really care. He says he wants to meet and talk. He offered me a job."

"Really?"

"Yeah."

Guaril regarded him in warm and brotherly concern.

"Can you—? Can you, y'know—*trust* him, man?"

"Old Max has been my friend since I was thirteen. Long before I ever committed to his Party. We've got our differences, but then, well, so did me 'n' my old man."

"Max is not your old man, Theo."

"No. No, I know that. But, still. I—"

"—He's gonna wanna talk about the pamphlets, no?"

"I suppose so."

"You—you want us to come with you?"

"Yeah, man," Siegfried smiled, sweet but tough, like a slightly-built but wiry Butcher or Bad-Boy gangster that, despite a delicate frame, packed a jackknife sharp as a shark's tooth in *ihre Gürtel* belt. "We can be your bodyguards. I've got at least twenty rolls of shit to fling at the guy, if he gives us any trouble."

"Naw, that's all right," Theo laughed. "I don't think he'll want me to bring anyone."

"What d'you think he'll say, brother?" Guaril asked.

Theo tilted his head in thought.

"I imagine he'll make me an offer, and I'll think about it. It could be good. . . . Maybe he's got a job with the Party to offer me."

"You won't take it, of course."

"Well, I'm not sure, y'know? I mean, if they let me in—let me into the hierarchy—I could, well, straighten things out, maybe. I don't like the Party's line, but there's a Left Opposition in Russia as it is, just like the Communist Workers' Party here. Maybe I could join that."

Guaril considered. His handsome acquaintance watched him as he mulled over the other boy's position. Siegfried chirped in ihren own sober, anarchist *Einspruch* objection, saying, "Can you really change the Party from *within*, Theo?"

"I dunno," Theo admitted. "I'm certainly doin' fuck all changin' it from the outside. I dunno. I'll see what Max has to say. Can't hurt to talk. . . . Don't worry. I ain't done this much just to sell out now, comrades."

They laughed. Of course, they said. They knew that. And well.

So, they bade him adieu, and let him traverse the city to his old workplace on the east harbour, a district he hadn't seen in more than a year.

It was much the same as it had been a year ago, dark, dismal, industrially grim. But there were new kinds of people there, now. There were Brownshirts by the dozens, keeping watch on the corners of the sad little streets.

A few of them looked askance at Theodor, recognizing him from the past. At least one of them had been one of the SPD clods who had called him a cocksucker, nearly two years before, when he wasn't even a cocksucker yet. The boy stared hard at Theo, recognizing him, and whispered something to his mates. They pointed at him and laughed. Theodor froze. Looking behind, he saw more Brownshirts coming down the little service road he'd just come down to get here. This little promontory between the rivers and the canal was isolated—there was nowhere to go. A dozen of them easily between the two groups, they beat the ground with their sticks as they began to charge him.

Someone shouted his name. He spun round, his fists raised. About twenty men were pouring out of the building to his side, waving sticks and clubs—*surrounding him!*

But they were KPD partisans! All with the same black leather caps with the red stars Theo still wore! They stared the Brownshirts down, waving their truncheons, roaring threats at the Nazis. The dozen stormtroopers turned almost instantly and fled, high-tailing it through the alleys to the side and back up the service road—clear out of the district!

The Communists all welcomed Theodor as if he were a long lost brother, which, to them, he was. They were warm, patting him on the back and shaking his hand, a few embracing him, calling "Theodor, Theodor, comrade." They asked after his love life—was he still seeing that cute little fraulein?—and extended their condolences about his father. Yes, they all seemed to know a lot about him. But, after the showdown with the Brownshirts, the whole thing was welcome, like coming back into the folds of an extended family. Then, Theodor saw Old Max standing there, a great smile beneath his grizzled moustache and arms outstretched as if to embrace a son.

"Comrade!" he called. "It's good to see ya!"

"Same here!" Theodor chuckled, relieved. "Same here."

"C'mon back here—to our little 'office.'"

The group went back into the building. It was a disused factory or warehouse, converted into office space. There were more than several businesses, or organizations, claiming the place, and the Spartakist corner was just one of many. A film company huddled in a corner, its doors plastered with fetishistic pornography, and down the way some kind of workingman's insurance mutual aid society advertised amidst a host of sickly, crippled old men, gathering on beat-up benches. It was an inauspicious start, Old Max laughed, taking his old friend up a flight of rickety stairs—but, then, they weren't paying rent, so what was the harm?

"How d'you keep it?" Theodor asked, as he was shown into a little bare office lit only by a bare light-bulb, swinging on a wire.

He sat down on a little stool before a desk behind which Max sat on another little stool. There were pictures up, of Lenin, of Trotsky, of Bukharin. Theo recognized them. These were, according to him and his friends, some of the principals of the new bureaucrat ruling class. But, he didn't say anything about this.

"We *took* it," Old Max answered the question. "In this district, it's *us* who make the law, comrade. You might say it's our little Soviet Socialist Republic, these docks. The city's thinking about giving the whole port away to some private company—put together by the Busch Wagon Company and those transport-agent parasites, Schenker & Co. They've chased all the businesses out of here in expectation of that sell-off. They're gonna give the whole waterfront away, this year or next, for a fifty-year lease to those money-grubbing bastards—all for less than the price of one year's rent! Ah, but what do their plans matter to us, comrade? Let 'em *try* and throw us out! We outnumber the Nazis in this district, the Bullen ignore us (because they know it'd cause 'em more trouble to oust us than leave us be), and the bosses don't dare close us down. They're *afraid*, comrade. We've got 'em on the *run!"*

They laughed. It seemed to Theo a little pat, this answer, a twinge of paranoia about the appearance of the KPD comrades, just in time, the office just waiting for them, cosy and rent-free. But Theodor ignored his paranoia with an effort. Max was all smiles and fond memories. They talked a little while, reminiscing. But, at length, Old Max came to his proposal.

"You know, comrade," he said, "that I respect you. I don't always *agree* with ya" (he laughed) "but I *do* respect ya. You've got a good mind, Theodor. You think like a natural dialectician, a natural materialist. Even what I've called your 'adventurism' was founded on good theoretical bases—even if I still maintain those bases are faulty. I'm not gonna admit to anything wrong I did or said, comrade. Even if I *am* addressing you in confidence, as comrade to comrade, as Party member to Party member, and can share with you my disagreements with the Party line. I *do* in fact take issue with you on a number of points, still. But, like a good comrade, a loyal comrade, I bow to the will of the majority in our Party—and that majority *understands* you."

Theo looked at him. It seemed a little too much to take. He knew well that the Party, even the relatively independent one in Germany, could not possibly agree with his contention that those hallowed figures on the wall behind Max were some kind of new ruling class. Theo let a few moments pass without saying anything. Then, he ventured, "They do, huh?"

Old Max smiled winningly.

"That's right, comrade. They do. Which enables me to offer you a position with the Party. A well-paid position. Theodor, we want you to become a full-time theoretician, to go to Russia, and debate your minority views."

Bullshit, Theo thought. In a politer way, he expressed his thought.

"No, no!" Old Max chuckled. "No, I'm absolutely in earnest! We want you to analyse the important problems affecting Germany today. And, Russia."

"What's the catch?"

"There's no *catch!* Honestly, don't ya think our friendship means anything? I've known you since you were first in the Spartakusbund—even *before!* I sent you to Russia when you were fifteen, as the youngest comrade of the Youth Brigade. You'd yet to completely break from the Social Democracy of your family, your father; but I knew you would—I *knew* you would be my comrade someday. Maybe you don't *agree* with me, Theodor—I don't agree with *you*—I'm actually opposed to this—I'll admit it!—but, still, I recognize the wisdom of Moscow, and I bow to it. As I say, maybe you don't *agree* with me—but surely, you *trust* me, a little?"

Old Max's eyes were so warm, so friendly, Theodor forgot all his fears. All right. Sure. The offer was genuine. But, what was the job, exactly? What would be his first task?

"Simple," Max said, pushing his stool a little closer to the desk. "Now, I've read your pamphlets, comrade. They're quite erudite, and I must say I don't fully grasp them, not totally. But then, I'm just an average working stiff, all told, and never had much of a head for theory. I—"

"—Oh, don't bullshit me, Max. You're one of the cleverest debaters I know. I mean—"

"—Debate, surely! I can argue a point! That's fighting—down in the trenches, dirty fighting. I can do that—and goddamn well! But, here's the difference, comrade: none o' what I said was *original.* I learned the arguments of the positions of the Party—and learned 'em *well!*—but, I didn't come up with any of them. These guys—"

—He pointed to the comrades behind him, the ones hallowed on the wall, in a matter-of-fact way, as if they were just workers like him, regular guys—

"—These guys, they came up with it all. What the Party has decided, Theodor, is that *you*, among all the many minds of young Deutschland—*you* have the capacity to come up with more! That's right, little brother; the student has surpassed the teacher. I gave you the theory. But, you used it as a base for *more* theory— more complex theory than I can even guess at. It's hard to admit that some young whipper-snapper can be so beyond me—it's hard, Theodor, but I'll do it. We're offering you to go to Moscow, and advise people like—*this!*"

He again motioned to Lenin, Trotsky, and Bukharin behind him, this time not matter-of-fact, but almost in awe. So swift, so inexplicable was the change, that Theodor had trouble really registering it. Max looked Theodor dead in the eye, as if to say with his eyes, *what else is there to say?*

And there seemed nothing else to say. Theodor knew he should jump at the chance. But he was a streetwise fellow, and as tempting as the offer was, he knew that precisely in its being tempting, there could be a trap in it all.

"So, what's my first assignment?" he asked again.

Old Max kept looking at him, his eyes wide, as if he himself were stunned by what he'd just told him, even still. Then, he shook himself out of it, and said, "Well, that's obvious, ain't it?"

"I'd say not."

"Well, Theodor. The reason they want you is what you said in your pamphlets."

"What I said in my pamphlets? But, what I said in my pamphlets—"

"—Shows the ability to reason as a true Marxist intellectual. That's why they want you."

"But, Max—I said everything I said to go against them! Why on earth would they want me?!"

"Easy, comrade. If you can tie something up, you can untie it. So, if you can reason out the flaws in your documents, using the same beautiful logic and argumentation that you employed to write them—well, then! Can't you see the service you'd be doing the Movement?"

"But, I'd never do that."

"Why not?! It was an exercise—a *brilliant* exercise—and it shows how formidable you are as a thinker. Why serve anarchists and bourgeois apologists with your mind, when you can serve the

People?"

"The 'people' is who I *was* serving, Max."

"No, no, no. No, comrade, no. It's easy to get lost in theory. Christ knows *I* get lost in it! The point is, none of us can refute you. Only *you* can refute you."

Theo laughed.

"Ya ain't serious," he chuckled aghast.

"I'm *dead* serious! Don't you know that the things you said in those pamphlets are exactly the kinda thing the bourgeoisie *need*? To *defeat* the workers' movement? You say there's some new class that's usurping the workers' movement."

"And that's exactly what I meant."

"But that's *fucked up*, man! You *can't* say that! If you destroy Russia, the only country in history that's survived the overthrow of the capitalist class, then what do workers have? What?—*Anarchy?!*"

Theo smiled. Softly, he said that it was precisely anarchists that helped him come up with all this stuff. So, *yes*. Anarchy was *exactly* where it was at.

Old Max looked at him incredulously. He honestly didn't seem even to understand who Theo was in that moment. He said, also softly, "Don't you know all the work that's gone against anarchy, Theodor? From Marx and Engels down to Luxemburg and Lenin? It's petty-bourgeois and utopian. It's anti-worker. It's what the reactionaries use against us. I was told that you had anarchy inside those pamphlets, but I refused to believe it. I couldn't imagine a comrade, a student of mine, could come up with something so unscientific and reckless and—and—and—*evil!*"

Theo narrowed his eyes.

"Evil?" he asked levelly.

Old Max had a look on his face which Theo had never seen. Something timid. Something of plain *fright*.

"Yes," he choked out his words. "Yes, Theodor. That's what led to the Kronstadt uprising—the thing that almost ruined the Soviet Union before it was even fully formed. That's what led to Makhno's banditry in the Ukraine—betraying the Red Army— betraying the Revolution—at its hour of gravest crisis!—with the White Armies marching almost to the suburbs of Moscow and Petrograd! It's lawlessness, chaos. It's the greatest danger to a revolution, worse even than reaction and the return of the rulers. Because it's the thing that doesn't inspire confidence in democracy.

And without democracy, there's—there's—"

Old Max just shook his head. Finally, he choked out in whisper—"There's **nothing!**"

"Well, Max," the young man said after a moment, "I never opposed democracy."

Old Max sighed deeply, as if restored to life.

"Thank Christ for that," he breathed. "Thank—aw, Christ! There's no Christ!—I *do* hope you still agree with *that* at least, right?"

Theodor laughed.

"I'm no *Christian*, comrade! What in Hell's name would make you think I was?"

"Well, after advocating anarchy, comrade, who knows? You *do* agree with democracy, then?"

"Well, of course! That's exactly what I mean. The Kronstadt sailors were protesting a lack of democracy. The bureaucracy is against democracy. That's all of our point."

"You—and the anarchists?"

"Me and my friends. My comrades. Some communists, some ultra-lefts, some anarchists and syndicalists, some autonomists. We all helped draft those pamphlets. It's a little strange to think that the Party would want me in their structure, Max. I mean, they *should* want all of us. 'Course, after 'Lenin's Levy,' so-called, where you guys let in even old Czarist cops into your 'Cheka'—your *secret police*—I can imagine they'll take anyone in who's useful to them."

"No! No, no! I'm not talking bourgeois democracy, and all that shit—!!"

"—Neither am I! I'm talking about the soviet system. The system of workers' councils, and peasants' councils, and soldiers' councils. Like Comrade Lenin said, back during the Revolution— all power to the soviets! All power to the democratic, spontaneous organs of workers' power! You might call that anarchy, Max, but I know some anarchists who wouldn't. But whether they would or not—that's what workers' power's all about. Nothing more, and nothing less. Any force that wants to destroy those organs of power, the organs formed by people coming together to run their own affairs—be it a Menshevik who wants a Constituent Assembly instead, or a Bolshevik who wants to steal the democracy away by imposing Party discipline on what had been free forums of free discussion—it's *all* anti-worker, comrade. That's what I said. I mean, that's what *we* said. And, maybe I do have it in me to write that out—but *Christ knows*, I won't. If that's the 'job' you have to offer me, man—***I ain't interested!"***

Old Max looked at him, his shock gradually coming to a renewed confidence, the confidence of hate.

"All right," he hissed, "all right—*comrade*—if you're gonna contribute to the fall of workers' democracy, in a power struggle between it, and *Nazism*—then what are you but a fucking Brownshirt yourself?! Goddammit—I tried to reason with you, Theodor—offer you something I'd *die* to do! But, if that's how you feel, I'm gonna change tacks. You wanna be an enemy of the Spartakusbund? Fine then—we'll *treat* you like one! You *will* stop spreading this fascist propaganda, or you *will* be sorry! Do I make myself clear?"

Theo looked at him.

"I'm not in your Party any more, Max. I ain't been in it for nearly a year. You can't threaten with me discipline. I'll write the truth as I see it, me and all my friends, whatever stripe of truth we come to—and *goddamn* your bureaucrat bosses! Look at 'em there, Max! Behind you, on your wall, like some fucking icons of some fucking feudal church! Lenin, who said that the working class will never get beyond 'trade-union consciousness,' and needs his Party intellectuals to *instruct* them on revolution, *lead* 'em and *push* 'em to it, like dumb, herded sheep!—despite the fact that it was *workers* who organized *themselves* into the soviets he's trying to emasculate—as far back as 1905—long before the Bolsheviks even supported 'em! And Trotsky, who built an army which conscripted the workers just like the fucking Czar's army did—with top-down leadership, himself the commander-in-chief—*and shot deserters!* And Bukharin—yeah, I know him, too, man. A guy who's trying to bring back fucking capitalism with his so-called 'New Economic Policy'—fucking *capitalism!* To save your sorry, bungled, mismanaged state! *That's* your goddamn Trinity! And damn me to Hell if I ever fucking bow to it!!"

Old Max just smiled.

"You've been warned," he pronounced, then got up swiftly and left the room. Theodor sat there a moment, breathing hard, trying to calm down. Then he got up, and made to leave the room. The door opened before he got there.

*"Theo! **Theo! THEODOR!!"***

The voice came through a long, dark, echoing tunnel. Theo opened his one eye, but couldn't open the other one; it was swollen shut. He was a bloody mess on the steps of the tenement where he lived. Katya was holding him, crying and cursing at what they'd done to him. Guaril and some of the anarchist kids were there, looking into the distance to a phalanx of retreating, raucously laughing men. There was a note pinned to Theo's cap, affixed there on his red star.

Katya read it, though she didn't want to. It said: "*Consider this your final warning, traitor—we* **know** *where you* **live.**"

"Who were those men?!" demanded Siegfried, half-looking to Guaril, half to the fleeing thugs, *ihre Fauste* raised, clenched and shaking, one *Faust* grabbing for *ihre Klappenmesser* jackknife.

Guaril knew. So did Katya.

They would have to leave Berlin.

Chapter 10

But, where could they go? Things all over Europe were mirroring the chaos of Berlin, truth be told. The workers' movement internationally was torn between the forces of reaction and the forces of freedom—and the reaction was winning on all fronts. Communist parties were entrenched in every country, now, and they were drugging the workers with the opiate vision that Russia was something they should aspire to. They had a powerful influence on the movement, now, its revolutionary tendencies, and there was still nobody, really, of a Marxian persuasion anyway, who was offering any criticism. Workers had that alternative, or some kind of right-wing Social Democratic one, to form their theory and world-view. It seemed hopeless.

But it wasn't, Katya assured. In France, there was a strong and growing contingent of anarchists and anarcho-syndicalists. Maybe they should go to Paris, she said, and join them.

There was also Spain. Guaril had only a few years ago left that country, his country, or at least, the country which bore him. There, since 1911, there had been the CNT, a confederation of anarchist unions, which had just recently officially rejected Russia's Bolshevism outright, to stand independent and free. Here, too, was a possibility.

For now, though, time was of the essence. There was no waiting around in Berlin for the Communists or the Brownshirts to beat them, or kill them, as they knew it was perfectly conceivable they might now. Theo was not about to retract his statements or those of his friends, and he could not possibly shut up about it all. The Workers' Movement needed the insight of the anarchists and the libertarians now, more than ever. The workers needed to know what Russia really was, and that they could not look to it any more as their model; the workers must realize that they need look no further than their own lands, their own tenements and factories and docks and farms. They needed the confidence to look nowhere but to their own mirror reflections. That is, if there was any hope at all for real revolution.

Katya still toyed with the idea of that farm in Bavaria. But Bavaria was increasingly in the thrall of the Nazis. That bucolic and beautiful place, where Katya had spent so many pleasant childhood summers in one of her family's summer homes, that place where just five years ago an independent, revolutionary council government had been declared—that place now, at the close of 1924, was the very stronghold of fascism in Germany. No commune they'd build together there could be assured of not being molested and persecuted, closed down, even burned to the ground by Bullen or fascist mobs. So, it was decided among them to quit Deutschland altogether, and take a tour of Europe by train, to see what they could see. Just hours after Theo had emerged from unconsciousness on their doorstep, they'd embarked.

"I've always had these dreams," Katya told her lovers in their first class compartment aboard a train heading to Antwerp, the first leg of their journey, "of trains. It's a little queer. I always think about them when I get on a train, that suddenly I'll be trapped, and lost, and all."

"I have such dreams," Guaril said wistfully, looking out their window, "too. They're archetypal, it seems to me. I have liked what I've read of Carl Jung, the Swiss psychologist, and his differing interpretations of dreams from Freud. He's made a kind of religion of dreams, reawakening in this dead Europe the spirituality available to everyone, every night. I myself have kept a journal of my dreams, every night over these past five years, and I've made scores of drawings and collages about them. . . . But, love, I think you can put too much into dreams, too, even if they *do* have significance. We're safe here . . ."

At the Belgian border, the first of many, they were checked for passports and visas and the customs people looked at their bags. But, everything was in order. They were not three fugitive revolutionaries, travelling incognito through hostile territory; or at least, they didn't really *feel* they were then. They were, rather, a rich girl and her two intimate friends taking a long holiday, living a blissful existence of pleasure, of love. Theo's wounds healed, over the next days and nights, as they journeyed west, then south, then west again, and the three made love in stopover hotels and in their bunks in the train compartment, late at night and in the middle of the day, in perfect privacy. They drank bottles upon bottles of the cheapest, sweetest champagne and sampled the best, driest caviar, ate oysters on the half-shell and artichokes drenched in butter. The taste of all this was new for each—for Theo and Guaril, surely, who had never tasted such fare—but, too, for Katya, who broke her vow not to eat the flesh of animals because of the greater thrill of defying religious convention, swallowing the roe and shell-fish in deep, satisfied sips. Their week a blaze of wet memories, they arrived at last in Paris.

Paris was beautiful. They walked its boulevards, took in its museums and its art galleries and its monuments and its many parks, and for a little while lost themselves in the welcoming hazes of late-night hotel rooms and early afternoon cafés. But, each of them knew this was all a fantasy, but the "honeymoon" of their well-consummated relationship; they'd have to come out of it sooner or later. As much as Katya liked the finer things, she was more than aware that privilege was an awful thing, and she hated it all in her way. Theo felt guilty for enjoying himself so much, though a little vacation was something he realized he needed, after the trauma of the betrayal by his old comrades. Max. How could he *do* that? After so much history between them, so close a friendship? How could boys he'd struggled alongside, planned demonstrations with, strikes, battled Brownshirts together—both with the Party's blessing and without it—closer than comrades, they'd been, for more than half a decade—how could they turn round and do *that?* The madness of the world was more than the madness of the individuals within it. It caught like a fever, a cancer, spreading through the ranks of humanity, making them into monsters—*one monster*—the monster of the Crowd. It made Theo almost reconsider his politics altogether, and sink into despair.

But, they rallied. They attended a conference of Syndicalists where they spoke with many workers and intellectuals, finding they were not at all alone in their disgust with what was going on. They'd mailed their pamphlets ahead of them to Ascona before boarding the train in Berlin, where Nadia and Sebastien awaited their wire when they arrived in Paris to send them on (so as to avoid any meddling at the borders whilst travelling on the trains). The pamphlets arrived in time, and they copied them and printed many more, Katya translating them into French and English, Theo into Russian, Guaril into Spanish, and all of them sharing the writings at the conference. They received and read much more in turn, finding their ideas had parallels in a host of languages. The idea of the New Class and the Revolution Betrayed was gaining ground and momentum, and it heartened the ménage.

The three met people at the conference who had gone to Russia, to a meeting of the International Congress of Red Trade Unions a few years back in Moscow. These syndicalists had pressured the Bolshevik government to release thirteen anarchists held in the austere Taganka prison, who were having a hunger strike to protest their imprisonment. The Taganka prison was infamous, long a Czarist prison for radicals of all stripes, from Bolsheviks to the Socialist-Revolutionaries who had helped form a coalition government with them in the first year of Soviet rule, but had now been banned and driven underground. Anarchists, too, had been held there; and some of the anarchists languishing there now were the same people who had been held there under the Czar— sometimes in the very same cells they'd spent years in, lowered into holes in the ground like graves—the Revolution, so recently risen, now buried alive. The pressure of the syndicalists in the Red Unions was actually enough to get all thirteen anarchists released during the Congress. (The prisoners, almost all of them, were deported from Russia shortly thereafter—one or two said to be living their exile right here in France.) It was heartening, this victory, proving that even in the now bankrupt, bureaucratized Red International, pressure could still be exerted by non-Bolsheviks within its most prized and guarded institutions. Theo and Katya and Guaril were impressed and soothed by these tales, giving them hope for the first time in forever.

There were lively discussions, less debates than the sharing of comradely views, in Paris and other cities and towns near it, and for a short few months, as 1924 became 1925, it seemed like some real progress was going to be made. Several organizations of syndicalists were being attempted, and there was a lot of confusion and in-fighting. But nearly all the workers themselves, whom in France were more syndicalist and anarchist-inclined than the workers of Germany or (certainly) Russia now, insisted on such things as "labour exchanges" (locally-controlled, autonomous union structures) retaining more power than any overarching organization. This safeguarded against the danger of centralism—even though the overarching structure of the General Union of Workers (the CGT) was openly syndicalist in theory and practice, and such danger seemed far off. Katya and Theo thought this was a very promising trend, as was the long-standing mandate amongst these folks that their unions would support no political party, nor would they accept the control of any. From what the ménage gathered, many workers in other countries were hanging on to the same freedom and autonomy in what they were doing, from Switzerland to Spain to Holland and Greece. Whilst famous men were arguing for "unity" amongst the syndicalist organizations, and jostling one another to "lead" them, there was an important insight a barber from Lyon told the trio late one night in a Paris cabaret after a demonstration.

"Unlike the commies," Gaston told them in a mixture of French and German, whilst giggling at the sultry, transvestite stripper doing her burlesque on the little stage, and doing something quite inventive with her tongue and the stem of a cherry, "we syndicalists have not proceeded from theory to practice. The commies began with a Manifesto, and then, based on that, recruited and built their great Parties and Internationals. But, with us, it wasn't *theorists* who made all us dumb oxen fight our fights; it was, rather, *we workers—we doers—*who worked and fought *first*—going back at least as far as the Commune! It was only later, much, *much later*, that any clever fellows made up a 'theory' of what we'd been doing—and then called it all 'Syndicalism.'"

He laughed and took a swig of rose-tinted beer. "You see the difference, *mes amis?* This is what you and your friends have been trying to say with your 'theories,' eh? That it must be the working people who must *do* something—just as it was workers who made the general strikes, and created the workers' councils, and created all the cooperatives—and get this, comrades!—*all on their own!* What you wish to tell us is that what is *organic* to the workers is *all* that can be trusted. And, I, *mes freres, ma soeur,* more than agree! Anything added, forced on top of it, separate from it—well, then! You've all called it a 'new class.' But I say, whatever it is, it is not workers. Because it is so *formal*, yes? So *proper*, and falsely clever. To Hell! I say, with the Internationals—*all of them!!* Rather, long live *us—the regular, mundane, **beautiful** People!!*"

Theo thought for the first time that all their theories weren't necessary, maybe. Maybe people would keep up what they'd always been trying to do—to live free and independent of all the formal people, the proper people, the rich aesthetes and their state and their photographic negative—the Party theorists of today. What working people did long before there were factories to organize—long before there were fields to be tilled. Every tribe of "primitive" people wanted to live freely and autonomously. Just as every peasant population, whenever they were left alone, organized themselves collectively and cooperatively. The Anabaptists throughout the Continent during the Reformation, the Diggers and Levellers during the English Civil War—and most recently, the peasants of the Ukraine, who kept the Russian Revolution alive for years after it had been crushed by the Communists in Petrograd and Moscow. The slaves had been fighting for freedom since Spartacus, Gaston intoned; and always, always, with the community and the individuals within it having ultimate say over their own lives, their own backyards. It was good to hear such sense. No complicated maths or professorial dissertations need be cited. It was, simply, common sense.

As the spring came in the midyear of the roaring decade, the government of France began to mobilize for war against the Riffians, a tribal group who had risen against French and Spanish colonial occupation in North Africa. Many people opposed this war, but they were mostly unaffiliated with organizations. The Social Democrats of France were, not surprisingly, a hundred percent behind the government's imperialistic adventure, and with some notable exceptions, even a lot of the Communist groups fell in line with it. These latter did not actively support the racism of France, especially not the left-wing of the main CP, the Left Opposition, who voiced a formal protest. But neither did most of the communists go out of their way to act against the war, not spending much effort to protest it beyond words and petitions—and this, to Katya and Theo and Guaril, was just as bad. Anarchists and syndicalists preached against the war against the Riffians and staged marches and demonstrations. But most of these forces were too busy with their own fights, strikes, boycotts, organizing slowdowns and sabotage and pushing for occupations of land and factories. It was actually in that same cabaret with Gaston and his flirty wife Marthe on a later visit there that the ménage first saw something written in opposition to the war. There, on the tables, amidst the wine and the candles and the overflowing ashtrays and the pornographic pictures of some of the prettier dancers, Guaril saw a flier for a group that called itself "the Surrealist Revolution."

"What's it say?" Theo squinted drunkenly, puffing on a hashish cigarette he shared with Katya, who was giggling with Marthe on her lap.

Guaril said nothing. He just smiled.

"Maybe," he murmured, "there's hope for this white race, after all . . ."

Later, in a hotel room, amidst a group of lovers they all met, raunchy and delicate as only the French could be, sleeping in little huddles on the carpets and in the armchairs, amidst drained bottles of green glass and burgundy, Guaril read the pamphlet aloud.

"'The white man is nothing but a corpse—a corpse who dumps his garbage under the natives' noses,'" he was smiling, giggling to himself that he and Marcus Garvey were not alone in the world. "This fellow, Paul Eluard, goes on to say there'll be a 'worldwide revolution overthrowing colonialism,' in which 'peoples of all colours will be absolutely free . . .'"

Civilisation, not just capitalism or communism, was the Ugliness these Surrealists wished to exorcise. And whilst Guaril read little else of their literature after that, he was happy others were working toward what he was beginning to see as inevitable. Katya had thought of "surrealism" as having to do with painting, perhaps with poetry, and music, maybe—the direction some isolated artists were going after Dada had dried up. But this articulation of it in a theoretical, political form was a new thing for her, as it was to both her boys and all their new friends in France. She felt very positive about it, and contributed an article to a renegade art broadside in praise of the Surrealist Movement, which was yet to fully flower.

By the beginning of summer, after the great Mayday marches and demonstrations, and other marches and demonstrations protesting the North African war, Katya and Theo and Guaril had done much to contribute to revolutionary theory and practice. They'd shared in the work against the war, and supported strikes and unions elsewhere in the country. They'd put together analyses of the colonial rebellion tying it to the workers' rebellions here in France, in Germany, in Russia and the Ukraine—whichever the form of government, the common people had common cause against it. They'd spread this message far and wide over the months of the spring.

But the heat from Berlin had followed them here, and this red heat was augmented by the old purplish and bluish flames of the capitalist order. Guaril was arrested on his way to the hotel they were staying at in Montmartre near the Seine, coming back from a meeting of young hustlers and ex-sailors who were trying to organize homeless prostitutes along the river to demand housing and an end to police harassment, and for over twenty-four hours neither Katya nor Theo knew what had happened to him. The gendarmes held him on a charge of lewdness or some such rot, and it turned out that he'd been in the company of a prostitute under a bridge who'd been known sometimes to work with the police. The young fellow had turned him in to save himself, and for a tense two days and nights, Theo and Katya wondered what might happen to their lover. Katya cashed in some jewellery and raised bail—a ridiculous amount of francs—and the trial promised to be lengthy and involved. A frame up.

"They hate us, you know," Guaril smiled without humour when Katya and Theo welcomed him into themselves in a frenzied reunion. The prostitute and the gendarmes were gadjo, of course, and it didn't take much to imagine the judge and prosecutors would be gadjo, too. It was time to leave France.

For a few days and nights, they hid out in a garret atop a dilapidated tenement near a coal yard on the Canal Saint-Denis, belonging to Marthe's deaf-mute, eccentric younger brother, a sculptor named Gilbert, a boy who would kiss your hand in greeting whether you were male or female. As he slept (and Gilbert slept for fourteen or twenty hours at a stretch), the trio planned where they might go next.

There were syndicalist movements in Switzerland, they knew, in Holland and Belgium and England, too. All of these places seemed good ones to run to. But in Spain, to the south, there'd been fighting in the streets between anarchist unionists and fascists, and there was a feeling that anarchy might actually come to the Iberian Peninsula, before anywhere else in Europe. The peasants in the countryside there, with or without any formal organizations, were said to be working out a collective, community-run economy. Though in just the earliest stages, it seemed these rebels were coming closer and closer to the ideals Katya, and now Theo and Guaril, too, held close to their heart. With the desire to fuck up the fascists, coupled with their increasing desire to claim a place, an island of Anarchy, for their own, it seemed in that sunny Parisian summer dawn that even sunnier climes to the south were beckoning.

Guaril, through his contacts with students at the University of Madrid, where he'd briefly matriculated before going on his years' long odyssey through gadjo Europa, found out that one of the French Surrealists, comrade to Paul Eluard and Andre Breton and the other writers, a fellow named Louis Aragon, was scheduled to lecture on surrealist solidarity with colonial uprisings in a hall on the campus towards the end of May. With the air charged with racist and counter-racist electricities, the Riffians still resisting French and Spanish imperialism just across the Mediterranean, Aragon's lecture seemed a great opportunity to meet and talk and connect with other Europeans who proudly aspired to "defeatism" for the project of White Domination.

On this note, the ménage a trios decided to take the two-hour train ride from Paris to La Havre, a grey, industrial port on the northern coast, going third class to avoid the eyes of the gendarmes who might know something about them and their predilections thus far to travel by first. From there, they booked passage, second class, on a steamship to Santander on the northern coast of Spain. Madrid was the destination after landing in Spain, whether by auto or train or horse-and-buggy—the trio cared not. From Madrid, they planned to go to Barcelona, the place of some of the recent fighting between the anarchists and the fascists, at least according to Marthe, who had cousins there.

Barcelona. The early place of Picasso before he'd gone to Madrid, and from there, the world. Picasso was a comrade, Guaril thought, though he would never meet him. It was brave Pablo who had first employed the African aesthetic in his art, his inspiration coming in the early 1900s from exhibitions of the masks of African tribal nations past and present, brought to exhibition in a Spanish museum. Though the curators doubtlessly thought the masks "exotic" and "primitive," Picasso was said to have told colleagues that he recognized the tremendous merit of the works, and worked through his own white fears of the foreign forms to forge a new aesthetic into European art, one which had yet to be fully appreciated more than a decade later. It was the beginning of the end of European art, Guaril intoned, the annihilation of the stifling tradition of centuries of whiteness. Modernity was, he smiled with confidence, the beginning of the decentralization of the Euro-North American influence on world affairs.

Guaril conceived of an art exhibition to show his own works to the public for the first time, works he'd been putting together in portfolio the past year, mostly as attempts to illustrate his dreams, and lately as cover art and illustrations for their salon's pamphlets. They were mixed media, mostly, images clipped from magazines and newspapers painted over and modified, so that they became archetypal, even such things as machinery and weaponry and manikins from department stores—all of these highly secular things, emblematic of the newest sciences and social trends, became subsumed into Guaril's overarching myth-making. Dream-sequences of modernity; Dada, asleep. Paris might have been the "proper" place to show it all, as Berlin might also have been, if the European cognoscenti were the ones he wished to create for. But Guaril wasn't interested in impressing such elites. Moreover, Guaril had not felt himself ready in Berlin, nor did he feel entirely ready yet in Paris. He felt that, though he was not a Spaniard, but a Gitano

Rom, first and last, he might well see it as fitting to start his public career in the nation of his birth. Especially considering the workers and peasants there were creating a situation where all their dreams might be realized. So, after their six month sojourn in Paris, they'd decided to trek down into Spain in the beginning of the summer of 1925.

It was to be the best, and the worst time in their lives.

Chapter 11

The threesome arrived in Madrid just hours before the talk at the university, the days and nights of travel by train and ship and flivver not noteworthy beyond the loving they shared along the way. The flivver was a beat-up Model T which they picked up third hand from an old con-artist for a few hundred francs, which the fellow took with a crooked smile and a broken French assurance that he'd done them a favour by not demanding pesetas. Guaril understood Spanish and French fluently, but let Katya do the talking, listening for any lies in the con-man's speech. There were far too many to isolate just one. The car literally began falling in pieces on the road, barely making it to the Madrid campus.

Guaril had been thinking seriously of the surrealists, and also the syndicalists, trying to make a fusion between the two, all under the umbrella of a Roma-centric politic. He spoke of translating some of what he'd read from the *Surrealist Revolution* papers in Paris into Spanish, and also into his rusty mother tongue. He thought to express his long-felt intuition that the plight of the Gypsies, one of the original "dark peoples" of Europe, who with the Jews seemed the locus for the genesis of European white racism, was intimately intermingled with surrealist and anarchist impulses to take down the whole monster of white civilisation. Theo sketched out ideas with him, as did Katya, scrambling to synthesize their thoughts into something they could hand out at Aragon's talk. They banged out a rough manifesto by the very morning on a typewriter as dilapidated as the car, printing a run of them on a roneograph machine in the basement of the five-hundred-year-old university's library, which they used under the false pretence of being graduate students of the School of Odontology. They found many eager hands grabbing them amongst the students in the lecture hall, smiles and scowls alike showing their words had great effect.

Others had come, a few Communists leafleting outside the lecture hall with copies of Lenin's polemics supporting the right of oppressed nations to rise against oppressor nations, and how nationalism was not one tendency, but rather two—dialectically opposing one another: the laudable urge to self-determination of oppressed peoples contrasted with the condemnable patriotism of the oppressor nation. The open-minded students snatched up these pamphlets along with the rest, and many probably thought that the surrealists, the anarchists, and the commies were all on the same side on things. Perhaps, in a less theoretical sense, they *were* on the same side. But Theo, particularly, was unimpressed by the Leninists, and he almost got into a fist-fight with one of them over the direction of the Comintern, the newly-forming revolutionist wing of the Red International.

Louis Aragon was poetic and stirring in his hour of attacking European colonialism, making it quite clear that he and his comrades supported any and all acts by the darker peoples against it. "First of all," he began stridently, yet matter-of-fact, "we shall **ruin** this civilisation!" (A wave of cheers rose and fell as his echoes rang through the lecture hall.) "This civilisation in which you are moulded like fossils in shale!" he went on. "Western world—you are condemned to death! We are the defeatists of Europe, so take care—or, rather, *laugh at us*. **We shall make a pact with all your enemies!"**

There were rousing cheers from the back of the vast hall, swelling up to the front. In that swell of shouts and applause, the French poet further declared: "And let far away America collapse with all its 'white houses'—in the midst of its absurd prohibitions!!"

The hour-long talk and the fierce debates which followed were a good christening to the new life in Spain. There were demonstrations in Madrid, marches and speeches, and as always, work: propaganda, of the word and the deed. In the next weeks, the ménage wandered all over the peninsula, getting every last inch out of the cheap flivver they'd bought, holding the pieces of it together with jury-rigged metal fittings and lengths of rope and even a few dozen well-placed rubber-bands, till they got to Barcelona and abandoned it in a scrapyard, and settled in for what they planned as a long and happy exile.

They settled in the Barrio Chino, a neighbourhood in Barcelona which at the time seemed more a place of foreigners than Spaniards. It was a dismal place, yet also very *alive*. Thieves and prostitutes and dealers of various underground substances abounded, along with beggars, clothed in silk shirts of yellow or green, beaten sneakers and blue denim trousers. These latter begged money in the square, at the marketplaces, saying over and over, with a dignity that was almost saintly, "*Por Dios, Por Dios . . .*"

Guaril spoke Spanish fluently, even more fluently than he knew French or German, and he was able to score them connections, things like marijuana and hashish and opium, things that helped the three ease their minds after hours of organizing and debating with fellow workers and fellow declassed intellectuals, who wandered among the slum dwellers of the barrio. Katya had a smattering of the language, and Theo too soon learnt a little. They enjoyed being revolutionaries in a place where revolution actually seemed more and more daily, nightly apparent. And, as foreigners, they attracted no more attention here than any of the others who abounded in the district.

They found rooms in a dilapidated tenement, on the fourth floor, a place of small but airy rooms, plastered white and almost sterile, but for the dirt. Living there was good in the next season. They connected with local artists and a host of anarchists, doing work with the CNT, avoiding the Communists, the Fascists, and the police. Theo contributed articles to anarchist and libertarian publications, translated by Guaril, and Katya made a small living for them by contributing to radical art magazines, particularly the newly-founded *AIZ—The Workers' Illustrated Magazine* in Germany, for which she contributed half a dozen articles under pseudonyms. She still had her connections with *Der Sturm* and *Die Aktion*, too (though the latter made a point of never paying their contributors a pfennig). With Guaril's help, she contributed, too, to Spanish publications, and her French was good enough to get an article or two in *La Revolution Surrealiste,* one anonymous article of particular pride in which she combined literary and artistic criticism with unedited pages from her own diaries, detailing sexual fantasies she considered too dark, too dangerous to indulge in anything but paper. Inspired by hundreds or perhaps thousands of hands and eyes unknown to her, scrutinising her dirtiest, most secret fantasies, their dirty fingers poking and pressing against her words, she almost managed to actualize these fantasies in the flesh, once or twice, despite the dangers to her body and soul—with strange men she enticed to follow her down dark alleyways—getting a fistful of pesetas and some gorgeous bruises to show for her night's work. And of course, she still had her stipend from her family, who did not approve, but could not really stop her from living the life she'd chosen.

Or, so she thought . . .

One day in early fall, a letter arrived from Katharina's father. Only the periodicals she corresponded with and a few far-flung comrades knew her address here, the trust fund lawyers who handled her stipend sending it to a bank far down the way. But this letter came straight to their tenement flat. It demanded, very forcefully and curtly, that she return to Germany at once. Her great aunt had finally lost her battle with her long illness, and there was an inheritance to work out. Though the tone of the letter was grim, even angry, the news itself was, she thought, positive. Her great aunt had suffered gravely with the consumption, had lost all but her mind over her last years, and those years numbered nearly ninety by the end; a full life, and now she felt no more pain. With her inheritance, Katya would be able to really strike out on her own, taking her friends with her, starting that communal, collective farm she'd always dreamt of. Here, in Spain, it seemed the peasants were already pushing for a collective form of living, though it would be probably years till this could actually grow into something of a mass movement. Katya, smiling, said they could pioneer the thing, she and Theo and Guaril, and her two best lovers enthusiastically agreed.

But, back to Berlin? This was a journey Theodor, anyway, could not yet contemplate. Old Max was still alive, and so was his Bolshevik rage. The KPD was gunning for him. Even here, hundreds of miles away, local Communists had gotten wind of the pamphlets and the ideas he'd acted as secretary for, penning down the collective thoughts of all their friends. The reactionaries were watching him and everyone he spoke or corresponded with. It was ugly. It wasn't enough to be watched by the police, who followed each of the three, as well as the intimate friends they made and lived with, not enough that the fascists were also aware of them. They also had to watch their back from the very comrades that, a few years before, would have risked their lives to defend Theodor from these.

"It's all about class," Theo said, confident, despite his broken Castilian in conversation with a few of their intimates over a late-night carafe of good, cheap, home-made Tinto de Verano. "The bourgeoisie hates us; the bureaucrats, too. They're in a death struggle, to reckon who's gonna run this world. It's like the American Civil War, or the Revolution there—slave-owners and slave-traders, working together to enslave the world, competing only in making hegemonic their one or another preferred form of slavery. It's only logical that each'd hate the slaves even more than each other. It's only logical they'd hate us. We ain't friends to either of 'em."

"The CNT brothers and sisters'll protect us, Theo," Guaril said, also with confidence. "They'll protect us all. We're their comrades—no matter our 'foreignness.' Stay here with us, while Katya goes back to Germany. Then, she'll come back, and we can quit Barcelona, find some place out in the countryside. What do you think, love?"

Katya smiled.

"That's right," she said in a Spanish-German patois all her own. "*Das-eso ist richtig-verdad*, Theo, *mein corazon, mi liebling*. You're safer here, probably, than any other place in Europe—anarchy's so strong here. And, despite all the Chekist crap, what the Bolsheviks know about us, we're still relatively anonymous here. I won't be gone long. Just a little while, maybe as little as a week or two. I'll sign the right bullshit papers, and I'll be almost a hundred million pre-war marks richer. Then, I'll come back and get you boys, and we'll see about that farm. Maybe near Andalusia. It's so warm, there, all the hoboes say . . ."

The few others in the apartment, sleepy and tipsy in the hour before the dawn, murmured their assent to this, and one woman, a dark, Arabesque beauty named Amina, who worked in a gun factory elsewhere in the city, stealing parts to build her own arsenal, nodded to Theodor, "*Verdad, mijo. Tu companjeros y companjeras—We all got yer back . . .*"

The boys saw their girl to the train station later that morning, along with some of their anarchist friends, and she waved prettily with a little silken handkerchief from a second class window, blowing them kisses, then fluttering her tongue in sweet obscenity. She waved her handkerchief to them till she was well out of sight, and Theo kept looking for minutes after the last shadow of the train faded into the horizon.

He would not see her again for nearly five years.

Chapter 12

Katharina had a strange feeling on the train by herself. She was plagued by a nasty déjà vu, in which things in the window, things in her cabin, even things like the scent of the air or the taste of her coffee reminded her uncannily of dreams she'd had. Her usual feelings about life were depressive feelings, phantom sadnesses and inexplicable gloom. But now, she was *scared.*

What was this phantom anxiety? Where was it coming from? As she crossed borders, tried to read or sleep, everything was fine. Yet, she could not shake herself of this feeling of dread. She even checked her ticket a few times, swearing that somehow, she'd gotten sidetracked and was on the wrong train.

But, no. Everything was perfectly all right. There was no reason for concern. She contented herself by writing letters and postcards to her lovers, to her comrades and friends, which she planned on mailing straight away when she arrived finally in Berlin. When at last she did arrive, she was greeted by her father and mother, who came in their chauffeured limousine. They began to take her to one of their villas in the countryside, west of Berlin.

They were taciturn, speaking little, though she hadn't seen them now for almost three years. But this wasn't entirely surprising. Even when she'd lived with them, many years ago now, they were never the most talkative of companions. Her mother would lecture; her father would grumble. That was the extent of it, really. They did not approve of her. But that was fine; she didn't approve of *them*, either.

She made a little small talk, or attempted to, asking after relatives and family friends, her elder brother and her younger brother and their proper little slips of wives, children on the way for one of them (she had to ask twice which one). To all this the mother responded courteously. The mother spoke of the new opera season in Berlin, how the director of the Berlin State Opera, that "edgy fellow" Herr Kleiber, was bringing out another of his "vanguard dreadfuls," some new piece by one of those expressionist chaps, Alban Berg.

"Oh, mummy, that sound's lovely. What's the opera called?"

"What was it, dear?" the mother asked her husband.

"Oh, who knows," he grumbled.

"—*Wozzeck!*" said the mother triumphantly. "Yes, yes.

149

That's what it's called. After some play written before the War. Or maybe it was during it, I can't say. D'you remember, dear?"

The father was silent. The limo drove down the roads of the countryside as the day grew more aged, and though Katharina had forgotten much of the particulars of this part of Germany, she began to realize as twilight came that they were not, in fact, heading for the family villa. Katharina questioned herself, trying to relax in the plush leather seats and putting out of her mind her renewed fear. Of course, she thought, they were going somewhere familiar. She just hadn't been out here for so long, she no longer recalled the particulars of the countryside.

But they came in sight of a building, then, that was quite definitely not the villa, nor anywhere else Katharina had known.

"Where are we going?" she demanded, watching the spires of what seemed almost a feudal castle, or Prussian military fortress, come clearer on the darkened horizon. To this, her father finally spoke.

"Katharina," he said sternly, "we know, and have known for a while, that your lifestyle and your health have not been the best. We've decided, for your own good, that you need to go to a place where you can get rest, and the help you need."

"What?! What the hell are you talking about?!"

"Don't curse at me, Katharina. That just shows your ill health. We've spoken to several specialists about your case, and it has been decided that you need help. So, we've decided to drive you out here, so that you can get the help you need."

Katya looked at her father, then her mother, then the forbidding building into whose courtyard they were entering. Several large men in white suits were waiting for them.

"This is preposterous!" she shouted. "I'm twenty-four years old! I'm an adult! You can't—you can't *commit* me!! I wanna talk to a lawyer!"

"You're sick, Katharina," the mother said, attempting to be soothing. "You always have been—even when you were a child. We've done all we can for you."

Katharina twisted round and and banged on the grill to the front seat, to get the chauffeur's attention.

"Wilhelm!" she shouted to him—"Wilhelm!—Turn this car around!!"

"Now, don't make this more difficult than it has to be, Katharina," the father said. "Go nicely with the gentlemen there.

It's a very pleasant place—you'll see. It's—"

"—*Fuck you! Fuck you both!!* I swear I'll see you both in *prison* for this!! You've no right—"

The car had stopped, and the white-frocked attendants were opening the door.

"Go quietly, Katharina," advised the father, as if he really did not care one way or another whether she did or not, edging away from her as she kicked and flailed at them. The attendants had already grabbed her by the arms.

They dragged her out of the car, kicking and screaming and protesting what was nothing more than a kidnapping. Desperately, she called to the chauffeur, who had been a servant of the family since Katharina was a small child. He looked on in impotent sympathy.

"Wilhelm!" she shouted. "Wilhelm!—**do** something!! *Please!!!*"

The servant, whom had always been the girl's friend, just shook his head sadly, and mouthed, "I'm sorry." Then, at his bosses' command, he spun the car around, and pulled away into the night.

The attendants were impervious to her shouts and curses—they seemed to have expected something like this. They pulled her arms back, and dragged her inside the foyer of the place, all sterile white and industrial green, where somebody shot her up with something in a syringe. The last thing Katya felt was her arms being forced into a straitjacket.

Then, all was blackness.

Chapter 13

A week went by, then another. Within minutes, it seemed, it was a whole month that Katya had been gone. Guaril told Theo not to worry; but in his heart he, too, was more than nervous. They both knew, or rather suspected, that Katya's parents were not the nicest people. Of course, she might not have even gotten to see them. The phalanx of enemies round Europe was gunning for Katya, too, as she'd been involved with Revolution for years, and anarchists, even more than other radicals, were friends to no government. Her class background, her money, had afforded her a little more protection from cops and other government scum than others. But she was, when all was said and done, as committed to their overthrow as any of her poorer comrades—and thus as much in danger.

After a month and a half waiting in Barcelona, Guaril and Theo began to talk openly of Katya's absence, and allowed themselves all the grim speculations they'd privately harboured and brooded over to come out into the open. Their friends, their comrades, were as poor and powerless as they were, and with them were soon evicted from their tenement flat, to wander the streets of the Barrio Chino. Amina, her comrades Guillermo and Manuel and Esmeralda—the men's main contacts with the CNT in Barcelona, who would vouch for them and who introduced them to others— were all spirited away one night, leaving Guaril and Theo stranded and alone. They wandered homeless, aimless through the Barrio over the next weeks, wondering at whom they could connect with in a place and time of increasing suspicion. Only the bums could be trusted; everyone richer—even many of the impoverished workers—seemed as capable of being informers as comrades, now. And without Amina and their other friends, many of those who might have been their comrades looked to the two foreigners in much the same way.

Where was Katya? Nobody knew. Doing a little detective work, Theo managed to get the home office of the shipping line Katya's family owned, and from that number, he was patched through to Katya's father's private secretary. But that cold woman told him that no information regarding Herr Von Rosen's daughter could be discussed with any of her former acquaintances.

"You gold-diggers are the reason she cracked up!" the woman spat, her contempt so strong she'd inadvertently let on to something she probably shouldn't have. "Good day!"

And there was silence.

Theo concluded, and Guaril agreed, that Katya was not in Berlin. She was somewhere else, some sanatorium somewhere, a virtual prison; she'd been disappeared. There were many madhouses, private ones, wealthy ones, scattered all over Europe. And Katya's family could have sent her to any one of these. It wouldn't have been the first time they'd done it to her; she'd spent nearly a year locked up, and might have stayed that way, were it not for her great aunt's intervention, and the old woman's spiriting her away from the hospital, the town, and even the country to take a long tour of the world. But now, her great aunt was dead, and there would be no one left who had the power or the inclination to save her again. Lost on some sickly sterile ward, Katya would be lost, and probably would come to lose her mind, truly, and then they would have a justification to keep her there forever.

Of course, there was another possibility, another, even grimmer thing to be gleaned from that cold bitch's term "cracked up." Katya might not even be alive now. She'd attempted suicide in her past, she'd told them before, as young as eleven years old. She was always just a step or two away from it. Maybe, Theo thought, shivering; maybe Katya had done the unthinkable.

Or, maybe they'd just said she had, and it was an assassination. Theo and Guaril both shivered, both wept, thinking on these last possibilities. Katya was lost to them, in any case.

"What are we gonna do?" Theo asked, his eyes wide and hopeless.

"I don't know," Guaril said soberly, looking away. They sat in the alley where they'd slept, near a group of beggars, filthy, sombre, silent in sleep. The winter was coming on, with its chills and wet mists, and they'd have to find some kind of shelter soon. They had no money. There was no work for foreigners, no work for Theo, who was lost in the lack of language, nor for Guaril, who was so obviously a Gitano, hated by employers and workers alike. Even the begging trade was difficult, since neither of them looked the part yet, and besides, which of the old ladies who went to market would spare a tuber or a fruit for them, a gypsy and a foreigner? Stealing came up, though neither boy was really a thief. They had a little moralism, it was true, but mostly it was daring and skill that they lacked. Being prostitutes could work, of course, while they still were clean and presentable, well-fed and healthy looking. But this, too, had its dangers, and it would be no time at all till they were as filthy and lice-ridden and starved as the young men sleeping beside them. All in all, it was very bleak.

But they had each other.

Theodor cried, and Guaril cried, and Theodor cried longer. Theo cheered Guaril when he fell into deep sadness, with the loving skills of tongue and lips and palms greased with Vaseline. But Guaril comforted Theo more often, taking upon himself the mantle of the elder, the daddy, the one who would stay strong. He comforted his boy in doorways, under arches, amidst the dustbins of the alleyways. Guaril hugged Theo so tight the smaller boy could not move. He pressed him against the rusty doors, and kissed him hard, enough to melt him in the darkness.

Theo yielded to Guaril, turning his neck in surrender to the older boy's ravening. Guaril bit at his pale flesh, reddening it where he bit, sucking traces of his life through myriad tiny pores, then leaving the mark to green and purple as he drew himself down.

Guaril ripped his boy's trousers from his legs, and tore away his underwear, throwing both into the alley's dust. He picked up his boy's legs and swung them over both his shoulders, pressing his back against the doors, the walls, pressing his own face into Theo's cock, sticking up stiff and pearly in almost fear of the hunger of his lover, straight into his daddy's hungry mouth, big and small between his teeth. Guaril devoured his boy's cock, reducing Theo to buttery, sighing cries, his tears welling up in gratitude and submission to his lover, washing away all regrets—at least for that hot, wondrous moment—over the memory of their other. When Theo screamed, high and long, surrendering his cum to Guaril's devouring, he let himself be flipped round and pressed face and chest against the rusty, iron doors, the dusty, graffiti-smeared walls. Loosening his own denim trousers, letting them drop to mid-thigh so his bronze ass rippled over his rough leather belt, Guaril eased his thick shaft between Theo's white cheeks and pumped him with his fullest devotion. Fear he pumped into Theodor; and anger he pumped, too, hard and heavy, for all their precarity, for all the injustice of the world, all its betrayals; with the burning need to have Theo, inside and out, he pumped him; and he fucked his willingness, and his passion, and at last his need to be the younger boy's God, to take care of him, to love him harder and longer than the world could hurt him. With all this, Guaril fucked Theo, till both of them came creamy and spurting and roaring hot in the lost alleys of the Barrio Chino.

One of them looked off to the side after they'd collapsed amidst the dustbins, and saw a man in a long coat stumbling away. They laughed at the voyeur they figured him for, and they realized they had in their affections a potential gig for themselves. They would fuck like this again, over and over in the alleys of Barcelona, and they would not mind the old men who'd invariably watch them. They'd easily ask and gladly take the old men's money, the two young, powerful pretty-boys. They'd fuck their fill of each other, giving the old men their show, taking their pesetas and giggling as the old ones waddled away, fumbling to right themselves for their long walks home, their middles slick and sticky with their voyeur's tribute to the boys they wished they could be, or be with in lieu of being, disappearing into nether regions beyond the young men's ken or caring.

The two men lived the next months very lean, very harsh, despite the joys they managed often to make of each other. They were arrested more than a few times, and spent some nights in the jails of Barcelona. They stole bread, wine, and other sundries from stores and shops, to keep themselves alive. They sold themselves, together or alone, to men cursed and ugly, till they became so cursed and ugly themselves that they could no longer score clients. They found themselves in little, narrow rooms in the cheapest transient hotels, condemned buildings barely standing near the waste dumps and the skid roads more derelict even than the Barrio Chino. Windowless, dark, stinking of urine and garlic and sweat, with only the weak light through the transoms near the absurdly high ceilings to help them pick the fleas off each other's bodies, to light their meagre meals after one or the other of them had gotten a turnip or a pepper from the housewives and grandmothers in the market. They knew the company of others, in the same discarded position as they, who with them huddled in those dark chambers through the winter months, listening to their tales of the riches of the smaller towns in Catalonia to the north and west, where things of value were said to just fall on the ground for the taking, and the bolder ones forced things to fall with a knife to the midnight throats of those who had them. Theodor could not bring himself to outright thuggery, to stealing from actual people with violent intent, however rich they were, though he tried his hand at pickpocketing once or thrice. Guaril found himself not as threatened by the idea of violence as things got hungrier, and though pretty still, in Theo's eyes, and in the eyes of what few intimates they had, with his curly black hair and now full beard, the spectacles he kept though they were now cracked and crooked on his face, Guaril came to be a fierce and brutal hunter. He found hapless bourgeois wandering too far from home into the derelict districts, who trusted his smile, flashing from the shadows, but offered too few pesetas for his kisses and his time; these men gave him what he wanted in the night.

As things became more and more desperate, some of the insanity of the world around them began to seep into Guaril's and Theo's own brains and innards, driving them crazy, too. Guaril began to speak spitefully of the gadjo, the non-Roma, excusing few from his critique. Even in his fellow bums, he saw the traces of prejudice, of fascism, of white arrogance which, he said, would sweep them, too, into the coming apocalypse of race war. There are more of us than them, he would say, even if he and Theo were now in Europe, the stronghold and citadel of the whites. Someday, Africa would march, like Hannibal once marched across the Alps—though this time, Carthage would *win* the Punic War.

Theo realized that even when Guaril was angry, he always said "us" to him. He considered Theo one of the Roma, or at least a brother or cousin to the Roma. And this honour he granted to various people along the way, for he'd loved many people, many gadjo, too, over the course of his life. It was not so much race in essence as it was in identity, self-chosen, that he saw as important. If a European divorced himself utterly from the white ideology that was in its ultimate form Nazism, then he or she could stand with the darker peoples as an ally. But whilst Theo pondered this politic, he also realized that Guaril was losing himself a little. There was something in claiming a culture which he'd never really had that tortured him, racked him with strangenesses he could not name. It was this very effort that kept him from losing his mind completely. But the contradiction was telling.

Guaril began to feel the calling of his Gitano past, however invented that past might actually have been. He became obsessed with finding a caravan, somewhere away from these cities, away from the gadjo civilisation which seemed more and more alien to him, and to Theodor, too. He began to ask around, amidst the bums and hustlers of the city as the winter came in earnest, for information about how to get out of it all. Few had any real ideas, even the sons and daughters of the peasants of the countryside, fresh from the fields. For not even they, who may well have had organic connections, family ties and ties of friendship, to places outside the Babylon of the cities—not even they could take Guaril where he wanted to go. Farmland was not the wilderness. Perhaps there was no wilderness left in Europe. But it was the wilds that Guaril longed to penetrate, get lost in.

For all his angers and hatreds and paranoias of the gadjo, Guaril's dreams were fulfilled in a man almost archetypal of the white world. A tall, Aryan vision was Wozzeck, a pale, icy-eyed loner of a Nordic, perhaps Scandinavian or even Icelandic lineage. He'd come to them the week before Christmas in one of the windowless, derelict hotel rooms where half a dozen lice-ridden wretches slept on mouldy mattresses on the floor. His hair was long and near-platinum, matted in curly clumps, his beard jutting nearly a foot from his chin, rusty ashen, like the tongue of some serpentine dragon lost to time. He smiled to them through a face of hard ashy leather, and it was uncertain whether he was twenty, or forty, or even sixty. He saw two fellows picking off each other's lice, and saw Guaril and Theodor itching.

"You wanna play a game?" he asked in a thickly-accented Catalan. The accent seemed akin to Finnish, though Guaril could not be sure.

"I got no money," Guaril answered.

"Oh, it costs nothing, friend. You ante only what you have crawling over your skin—again, for it is free."

Theodor answered, drunk on cheap plonk and hunger, in a butchered Catalan.

"Sure," he laughed, "I'm in."

"Here."

The fellow pulled a dirty, empty jar from his ragged cloak, and set it down on the floor.

"Here," he said again, and reached into his hair, and pulled out a flea. He set it down in the jar, and grinned, "Now, you, huh?"

Theodor laughed again, and picked out a flea from his armpit. He put it in the jar, and the queer fellow grinned and screwed on a lid punctured with tiny holes like a salt cellar.

"Now," he smiled, holding the jar up between them, "let's see which of our little fellas wins, huh?"

The room came alive then, gathering round the jar, as the two tiny creatures attacked one another, brutally tearing into one another, jumping evasively, the bums laying bets of bits of clothing or peppers or the dregs of wine bottles to see which of the creatures would triumph in what became a battle to the death. It took fully ten minutes for a victor to emerge, and by the time it did, it was so maimed it staggered round and died, too.

The odd man encouraged everyone to try his little game, and it amused the young fellows for the better part of the night. Guaril laughed, and Theodor, and soon the fellow had begun to talk with them about getting out of the city.

"Wozzeck," the fellow called himself, a word in the German and also the Polish suggesting "Jedermann—Everyman." His lineage, his origins, his mother tongue, all were mysteries, and they remained so as he led the two travellers out of the city, showing them how to jump aboard a mule-drawn carriage and hide amidst the straw, riding it unseen until the dawn, when they jumped down into a ditch by the side of a barren olive grove. Though none could say what his past was, Wozzeck seemed to know intimately what Guaril's and Theodor's were, naming by their accents every place they'd travelled, guessing how long they'd stayed. He promised to give Guaril what he'd been begging the universe for the whole season: he said he knew the way to a Gitano caravan, and would take them there.

They spoke the Catalan none of them knew well. For Wozzeck spoke no German, no French, little Spanish; and neither Guaril nor Theodor could figure the Aryan's true tongue, the man offering no help in dispelling the mystery. They spoke brokenly, employing awkward idioms none knew really well, to try to convey the meanings of things, never knowing for certain whether any were truly understood. Wozzeck might well have known German or Polish, Swiss or Swedish or Finnish—his name, after all, was taken from a language Theodor and Guaril knew well. But he grinned as if an impossibly alien, barbarian brute from some savage, ancient epoch, and refused the colonization of these newer tongues. If it weren't for his pallor and stature, Guaril might have figured him for a Basque, whose tongue was said to be the most ancient of any spoken in Europe, unrelated to any of the tongues spoken from Gaul to India—for when the man spoke to himself, whistling through his teeth and spitting, his utterances conformed to no cadence Guaril knew. Theo himself wondered whether the fellow traced his lineage to the aboriginal reindeer-herders called by many "the Laplanders"—or the *Sami,* as they called themselves—the last of the indigenous peoples in long-cultivated Europe; for he knew well the ways of the wild, knew what to hunt and what to gather as they made their way through wilder and wilder climes. Whatever and whoever Wozzeck was, he was destined never to be pinned down by the two wanderers; his origins, as his intentions, were to remain a mystery forever.

In the broken tongue in which each of the three was equal in his ignorance, they spoke of the world. Guaril tried to tell him of his views on race, Theo his views on class, stumbling to translate their jargons in the butchered patois they were forced to speak. Wozzeck grinned and nodded in the camp fire light as they neared the Pyrenees, taking a sip from the thin stew he'd brewed from wild plants and roots he'd found over the day's trek through the hilly countryside, then passing the dented, tarnished copper pot of it to his companions.

"This world," he said, grinning wildly so his canines flashed in the firelight, "is too big for an idea, huh? *Any* idea. You sees 'em, huh?—the beastie all 'round us? And, the tree and the grass and the rock? They gots no 'idea.' They's too dumb, huh? But—" (he grinned sharply) "—they's *smart*, too—huh? For being so dumb?? Pretty soon—you give it time—maybe next year, maybe next twenty year, maybe next hundred—and we all be dumb like them. *If* we smart enough!"

He laughed a big, Viking laugh.

"'Fore then," he continued, "we all gonna get real, *real* clever. There gonna be clevers who gonna build big weapon, gonna breed big disease, gonna brew big poison. There gonna be clevers who gonna explain all that, and sells it to everybody, huh?—make 'em think they gots to have these big uglies, so they ain't dumb, like the dumb beastie, who ain't *clever* enough to build 'n' breed 'n' brew them big thing. And ain't y'all gonna smile and laugh, then, huh? Ain't y'all gonna be so *proud* o' us clever man-beastie, what ain't them dumb-beastie?? Oh, it'll be a *riot*, huh?! A big, *real* funny joke!—to giggle wit' them giggler!! Most all of 'em'll be giggling their way to their grave, huh? And, me? I'll be out here, giggling with the tree. All lonesome, me, out here with the tree, the rock and the dumb beastie. But, when all them clevers in the cities've laughed they breaths out, and lay like—like *stinking corpses*, huh?!—I'll be out here, still a-breathin'. . ."

Guaril and Theodor figured the big Viking queer and crazed, and they just laughed. Both of them saw apocalypses in the future, class wars and race wars and the fall of civilisation; both had hopes for something better rising like a phoenix from the wreckage and the ash. Wozzeck, though, put no stock in the new formulas or the old ones. He saw no hope in the apocalypse; nor was he downcast. He had no solidarity with a people or a class, a nation or a politic. Wozzeck was an animal. Alone, in the jungle. That was the only sense, he hinted. And whether anyone agreed with him or no, he giggled with self-assurance that they'd all end up in the jungle with him, when their great machines fell to rust and ruin, their cleverness delivering them to stupidity through following cleverness' own course. They'd clever themselves into mindlessness, he laughed brokenly, waving his hands and making signs to help him argue: Y'all will make profitable industries out of killing each other, till your facts and figures 'come so convoluted, nobody'll even understand the mess in their heads! Then, people'll return to kinder, gentler stupidity—which is their only hope. You'll all be back in the jungle, if you're clever enough to be dumb, Wozzeck giggled over and over, straining the words almost beyond sense. And if y'all don't make it—all of you clevers, dying and drowning in your clever convolutions—the Viking Wozzeck could care less! He'd be giggling with the rocks and the squirrels and the mosses and the mosquitoes as the great skyscraper ziggurats tumbled and the unsinkable Titanics sank!

"What are you sayin', man?" Guaril asked finally, laughing less now as the night grew darker before the dawn.

"What I say," the vagabond giggled, "is he what giggle last, giggle best. Huh? Huh??"

They nodded to him, and joined his laughter, softly, soberly. Then, they all fell asleep under the stars.

As the chill, misty winter waned finally in the ancient Iberian forests, in the shadow of the ancient mountain range, Wozzeck was true to his word. He brought the two men to a Gitano encampment, and hailed the gypsies there in fluent Romani, as if he knew them. Then he prepared to leave his two erstwhile companions behind with them there.

"How can I thank you, my brother?" Guaril asked Wozzeck in the Romani tongue he'd not known the fellow spoke all these weeks.

Wozzeck smiled, a trace of grinning evil in his icy blue eyes.

"You know it," he returned, in butchered Catalan, "the

price of the Ages, huh?"

"What?"

"Like that Bard say, the price of Wisdom, the clevers' tithe. I want from you, a *pound of flesh.*"

Guaril laughed, nervously squinting.

"I beg your pardon?"

Wozzeck grabbed Guaril's arm.

"From **here**, huh?" Wozzeck said, licking his lips over his formidable canines. "Cut me some of your flesh—and it makes good *meal* for Wozzeck!"

Guaril pulled his arm away.

"Won't pay tithe?" Wozzeck grinned evilly.

"Well—no! No, man! I can't—do that!!"

"Oh, no? You refuse fate, then, *Gwaaa-rrrrilll*?"

"Well, I—I—"

Wozzeck did something even odder, then. He whistled through his teeth and spit, once to one side of Guaril, then to the other side, then danced round him, spitting, counter-clockwise, his arms and legs all jutting out at weird angles. Then, he looked him dead in his dark eyes and said, "If you no pay me my pound of flesh now, you'll pay it later, *myyy broo-therr.* Ha ha!! You'll pay it, to **sommme-onnne ellssse!!**"

"Who the fuck are you, Wozzeck?!" Theodor demanded, his fists clenching, his pale face reddening.

Wozzeck looked at him.

"You owe me, too," he giggled. "You, *half pound.*"

"*Who the fuck are you?!*"

Wozzeck looked in stony seriousness, though his grin was wide.

"Wozzeck, huh?" he said. "Everyman, huh? *Ev-er-y Ma-an. Jeder Mann*—huh? Huh?!"

He leaned down to squint into both men's faces. He whispered:

"*Jeder Mann ist Gott . . .*"

And then, he traipsed off, losing himself in the woods. They never saw the stranger again.

The Gitano camp the stranger had helped them find was alive in the twilit forest in the foothills before the mountains, with the music of violins and vihuelas and young voices, male and female. Guaril declared right then they were "our people." He really wanted to talk with them, to share with them, perhaps even to join them on the road. And he wanted his Theodor to come along. Guaril hailed an old man there in the tongue he'd known as a boy, a tongue he'd had to relearn, later, as a man. Despite his best efforts, he spoke the tongue with an accent, a strange, gadjo accent, part Spanish, part German, part French, part Dutch, part Swiss—a little part of every tongue he'd learnt thereafter, during his long wandering through the world. But the old man spoke back to him, as Guaril explained himself. They spoke a quarter hour before anybody else in the camp noticed the two strangers' presence. Most all of them were sitting together, watching the dancers and singers and musicians perform, wondering at the *duende*, the magic, of their music and their dancing.

The old man just laughed at Guaril's bemusement at Wozzeck, saying he knew the crazy gadjo beast from way, way back. He never knew how the Viking could locate the caravan, over its wanderings through the north country near the Pyrenees; but he always could find them when he wanted to. Maybe he knew how to track them, the old man surmised. Ah, that Wozzeck was a wild one, the fellow said, and Guaril concurred—far more worriedly than the old man. But, not to worry, the old fellow said. He was as harmless as he was dangerous.

"A beast," the old fellow said. "A hunted, as much as a huntsman . . ."

"Yes, sir," Guaril said, "but he—he tried to *eat* me!"

"Yeah, he does that. . . . Tell me, boy, you like the music?"

Theodor was watching the dancing young people, and the old ones playing the violins and cimbaloms and all. His face smiled brightly, like the youngest child.

" . . . Your pal seems to."

"Oh—oh, yes, sir. We both love it. The *duende—the duende!*"

"Yea, it's somethin'. Tell me, you ever heard the story of how the violin was made?"

Guaril smiled, feeling as if he'd just been offered some down-home cooking he'd longed all his life to sample. He sat down beside Theo, as the old man sat beside him, on a log by the dancers.

"Why, no, sir. I've not heard it. Would you—would you tell it to me?"

"Yeah, then . . . Yeah, I'll tell ya . . . Seems there was this pretty lass, Mara was her name. And she was in love with this huntsman, who never gave her the eye—never even answered her when she called to him in the forest. . . . So, she goes to the Devil, o'course, and she offers Him her blood, for a favour . . . Devil's a tricky ol' bastard, though—ain't he, now? . . . Gets 'er to give 'im her father and mother, her brothers and her sisters, all for a chance to get that huntsman to look into the Devil's Mirror. . . . Well, he looks, and she looks, o'course . . . and then they're both fucked, y'see? . . . But the Devil tells Mara, 'I'm gonna make yer brothers and sisters into strings, each one thinner than the first. . . . And, I'm gonna make yer daddy into a body—the body of the fiddle, y'see? . . . And yer mummy, with 'er pretty hair—she, I'll make into a horsehair fiddlestick.' . . . And then, that ol' fucker, He played that violin, and enticed that aloof ol' huntsman to come to Mara, and he did, and they were happy, till . . . till, one day, the ol' Devil said, 'Now— *WORSHIP ME!!*—*For I'm Your **LORD!**'* . . . And He carried 'em both off, y'see, 'cause He had their blood, 'n' their reflections in that mirror, 'n' all . . . And then, y'know, a Gypsy came, and found that fiddle the Devil left there on the forest floor, and the poor ol' Gitano, he picks it up and plays it—and that old man, why! he can make Mara and the huntsman sing and cry, any time he wills it!"

Guaril laughed with the man, though he didn't really get what the story meant. He wondered if it meant anything, or whether the odd old fellow just liked to talk to hear himself talk. The fellow leaned in then, just as the dancing and the violins and the *duende* reached a crescendo, and whispered—"*You're a little like Mara, eh boy? Pining, ya are, for that huntsman?? **Careful**, now—Be sure as ya don't give away yer blood for it! Otherwise, **they'll make ya sing and cry . . .**"*

And Guaril still didn't know what the old man meant.

He looked round him. The forest was thick, and the vista of the mountains through the canopy caught the alpenglow of a late sunset. The camp around him and Theo was just a circle of a half dozen wagons in a clearing, all brightly, even garishly coloured and decorated, of the most vivid reds and purples and golds. Everything gave the impression of being somehow touched by magic, lilting, mysterious and beautiful. Yet, to Theo, who was not unkind in his appreciation of these people and their few possessions, the camp was what it was: a relic, an anachronism, of incredible poverty and insecurity. Most Gitanos in Spain, as most Roma everywhere, were long settled down—mostly in the ghettos and slums of the gadjo cities and towns round Europe. These thirty-odd souls had resisted that domestication, had clung to their nomadic life of times past in defiance of the Modern Age. The caravan was on the run, as it had been since before the young women and young men who were dancing, delicate with Romani beauty, not sixteen or seventeen years old yet, had even been born. They'd been on the run that long, fleeing the Spanish gadjo authorities, which had, in closed rooms in some city hall somewhere, declared their caravan illegal, and all caravans like it in Spanish lands. These people were not criminals, not in their own minds. For them, this caravan was the whole world, and they, like some latter-day Israelites, were wandering through a hostile desert, as their oldest members had been doing since their great grandparents were little babies, and longer. All through the long legends of their people, they'd known the wandering, the feeling of being foreign in hostile lands, like that exodus in that great gadjo book they'd never read. They could not read; the elders had never known schooling, and they'd collectively decided to keep their young ones from learning any of the gadjo ways, too. That way, the young would not leave them.

Guaril had left. But now, he had returned. And the Roma, the Gitano people of the caravan, quelled their suspicions of him and his gadjo friend, for he was saying how ugly was the world he'd been forced into, being stolen as a boy from a caravan much like this one, so, so long ago. Guaril told them, and they listened, and in his talk was a confirmation of all their fears and hates. They knew the gadjo as bullies and thugs, who dressed in the same silly uniforms and thus thought themselves something other than bullies and thugs. But the Gitanos had no illusions about them. They were monsters, simply, and those in the caravan were as proud not to be a part of them as they themselves seemed proud not to be Gitano.

Though they did not read, they had music, they had legends, and they had many skills. Generations of peasants had waited for them to come through in their long, roundabout journeys, to fix things round their farms, to sell them utensils and pots and pans of tin and copper they'd crafted whilst journeying, to trade jewellery of silver and gold the artists amongst them fashioned. But with modernity, factories now made those things, tradesmen now mended; the travelling, tinkering souls had been slowly, steadily replaced. But they were still sufficient unto themselves. Guaril looked on, sitting on an old log, to the pulsing dances which had with Moorish and Jewish dances once syncretised Flamenco, back in the 1500s, when each of these communities had found common cause in their common lot. The Most Catholic King Ferdinand and Queen Isabella of the Unholy Reconquista, and all the refined thugs of gadjo imperialism since them, had made of the Iberian Peninsula a place where none but the white could survive. True, they did not as often call themselves "white" as their fellow gadjo in the northern countries. But they acted in the same way toward those whom they considered not their kind as all the other monsters of Europe had. Guaril talked about this, about the learning he'd managed through universities and through self-taught history, reading between the lines of the official histories of Spain, France, Holland, Switzerland, Germany—to find this self-same story, repeated over and over and over. The people of this land, and all the lands the wanderers trekked through, were alike in that they defined themselves as normal, as conforming to some ideal which, though they rarely stated it in words (though the Nazis had an idea of it, with their blonde-haired, blue-eyed, perennially healthy and invincibly strong Aryan archetype), always defined them. And those who did not fit, they cast into the nether regions of their world, the periphery of their towns, the back-country wastes, the abyss—if they suffered them to live at all. And there was a time coming, Guaril prophesied, when these poor people would have to arm themselves, and fight.

"Otherwise," Guaril promised, "it'll be the end of us all."

The attitude of the Gitano boys and girls was one open to Guaril's militancy, though each of them wondered openly how they could possibly win such a battle. The gadjo were many, many. They had governments, armies, many allies. And we? We are but this caravan, and the other little caravans scratching a living over this continent. All the others of us have long succumbed to them, wasting away in their back-alley barrios, starving, shivering, drowning in the sludge backing up from their sewers. Even if we could get together, how could we possibly win?

"I'd rather die on my feet," Guaril said sagely, "than live on my knees."

The old people were more reticent. This kind of talk, Guaril's kind of talk, was destined for failure. Plus, it was foreign to them. Sure, you could rip off a gadjo, or even kill one, in defending yourself. But, to coordinate some kind of "army"? This was gadjo thinking, that "mass movement" kind of crap that never included any Roma anyway. It was the order of the day outside this caravan; surely, they could admit to that. But it wasn't *our way*. Better to live well, whilst we still can, than commit mass suicide in some

Pyrrhic gesture of desperation. This is what the elders said.

"You've been reading too many books, boy," laughed the old man who had originally befriended them when they'd first come into camp in the dusk of the night before. His name, he shared despite his avuncular mocking of the young hothead, was "Fonso." He told Guaril he liked him, in a way that reminded the younger, erstwhile Gitano of his own father. He put his arm round Guaril, and whispered something in his ear.

It was dawn now, and the camp was picking up their sundries to move on. Guaril wanted to come along.

"What?" Theodor said.

"I wanna come with, brother," Guaril said. "Fonso told me we could come. He's a widower, childless; we could help him, you know? and he'd let us stay with him in his wagon . . . Come along with me! They'll all have you." (He smiled.) "Just, you must learn to forget your gadjo lingo, and take up our tongue. Don't worry; I'll teach you. Pretty soon, you'll forget you spoke anything else. You'll 'acculturate,' as I once did to your society. And then, you'll marry some pretty Romani girl here, and your blood and mine will be one."

Theodor was more than tempted. There was something in all this that was akin to Katya's dream of getting that farm in Bavaria, or Andalusia, or some other such wondrous, foreign bucolic place, that commune where they could build their own ideal society, whether society at large ever changed for the better or no. It wasn't sticking your head in the sand—it was *living*, freely and truly, the best thing to do in a world gone mad.

But, what about Katya?

"She's dead to us, man," Guaril said, his eyes tearing over, but his face steady. "We gotta face that. We'll never see 'er again."

"I can't accept that," Theo said. "I gotta get back, brother. I gotta get back to Germany, and look for 'er."

"What if she's dead, Theo? What if that secretary meant she finally killed herself?"

"Why would she do that?!"

"You know and I know why. There's really no reason to go on in this world at all. It's not right for you to ask her why she killed herself. Rather, it's as telling a question to ask you why you still live."

Theodor looked at him, and wondered then of his destiny. Should he stay with Guaril here? In these forests, there were no communists, no fascists, no cops. In these forests, too, there was no hope for political anarchy. Rather, there was a natural anarchy, a natural egalitarianism and sharing here, which was as great a hope as any of the dreams dreamt back in Barcelona or Berlin. It was small-scale, but true. Whereas the world outside, with its syndicalism and its anarchism, with all the forces arrayed against these, seemed a hopeless thing. Theodor's father's prophesy merged into Guaril's. It was not class which would be the determining factor in this already dark century. It was, as the American Negro W.E.B. Du Bois had said in the last years, a question of the colour line. And the forces were gathering on both sides. Colonial rebellions, movements of liberation, all over the world, on the one hand; and, round here, the rise of fascism. The White Race, not content to rule in just that name, was making itself "purer" by purging itself of its undesirables. The Jews, the Roma, the queers, the mentally ill, the physically disabled—all of these were going to be separated from the rest, to make the white race *stronger.* And the battle they were gearing up for, that they were making themselves stronger for, was a final attempt at domination, slavery, and ultimately, extermination. The Nazis would take Deutschland. The eugenicists round the world would purify the Aryan race—be it Teutonic or Anglo-Saxon—on either side of the great ocean, these purists had their allies. And meanwhile, the darker peoples were rising . . .

Yet, Theodor still thought of class, struggled with a class science, which could enlighten people to take control of this beast called civilisation. He wanted to be sane. Yet, he knew that his metaphor, even if it was in his mind not a metaphor, but *reality*—his metaphor, of class struggle, would not be the dominant one, would not be the one that people would be moved by in the mad poetry of coming history. Guaril was right, he thought. And nobody thought quite like Guaril. But Theo knew nobody thought quite like himself, either. They were declassed intellectuals, and as such rubbed elbows with all the other rejects of society. They had been beggars, they had been thieves. They had been prostitutes, they had been revolutionaries. But what did it all matter now?

Theo decided to accept the hospitality of his hosts, and stay and love his friend, all the while pining for the memory of his other. They travelled the last of the winter of early 1926 in a world of their own, through the high passes of the Pyrenees, few and far between, with the Gitano caravan. Then, as spring warmed the land, they crossed into France.

They went over a bridge, many bridges over sheer cliffs and ravines and raging rivers and steaming, sulphurous hot springs. And each time they crossed a bridge, Theo and Guaril were told the same story by Fonso, as they sat with him in the front of his gilded purple wagon, the lead wagon, taking turns driving his horses. It was a tale that had been with the caravan for many years, told by lost great grandfather's grandmothers. Maybe it came all the way from Transylvania, or Turkey, or Egypt; maybe it hearkened back to the lost Indian Subcontinent, the genesis of the Romani people, long lost in misty legend and obscurity.

"There was a bridge-builder," Fonso would always say, "named Manoli—the eldest of twelve brothers, y'know. . . . He and his brothers shared the same boss-lady, who carried a tray on her head, and a babe in her arms . . . Now, Manoli had a wife, Lenga, and she dropped a ring in the water where the bridge spanned, one half high, one half low. And she bade her husband—'Go! And fetch my ring from the waters!' . . . And Manoli said, 'Yea, my wife, I'll go fetch it.' . . . And so he reached for it, and fell in. And then he was made the talisman—the cornerstone, the centre pylon—for that bridge he built. . . . Now, of that boss-lady, Manoli told God to tell the winds from his death, that it should blow off that boss-bitch's tray from her head in front of Lenga . . . And then, Lenga saw the snake, arising from that head—? Yea, yea, I think that's how she goes. Let's see, now . . . Yes, and there were two men—no, it was three . . . And the last one told Lenga that she'd drown, too, like her husband, y'see. . . . And she cried—'But my kids! My kids!!'— Y'see, she saw that snake . . . And then, she drowned, too. . . . I believe the two of 'em are in that bridge to this very day . . ."

Theo was completely lost every time Fonso spoke these words, spoken in Spanish or Catalan or Romani depending on the old man's mood, words that were translated by Guaril into German to the point where Theo could almost recite them after their time on the road. But, though the words of the story were varied every time, the story's forms changing at the old man's whim, the words never made any more sense to Theo than the last times the old man told them. Guaril pondered the old tale, fragmentary as it was, realizing Fonso was always laughing about it, that he might have been drunk, or senile, or just soft in the head, and that he didn't really remember the old tale his grandfather's great grandmother had told him. But Guaril also knew that, like all the Romani culture around him, it was all lost, and found, all at once; and, too, it was always to him a stranger and a foreigner—no matter how familiar the once-and-again gypsy was with the tale.

But this time, Fonso said something else, as they crossed what seemed their last bridge into France. He extracted a moral for the obscure remembrance.

"Y'see, boys," Fonso said, grandly and vaguely, his near-sighted eyes fixed on the far horizon, "Manoli is a bridge-maker. Roma were always the bridge-makers where this tale comes from—back east of us, and long ago—in Wallachia, er Greece, er Turkey, maybe—wherever it was . . . And sometimes, the bridge-carpenters would bury their wives in the pylons, to *bless* the undertaking, yeah? . . . And, sometimes, well, he'd just have to bury *himself.* . . . It's a dirty business, buildin' bridges, boys. . . . Sometimes—nay, *all the times*—you gotta stand, breast-deep in that river, 'n' look for that wedding ring dropped so careless in the waters. Sometimes—nay, *all the times*—you gotta give up your life, 'n' the life o' all you care about, to make that bridge have a *heart* . . ."

When they crossed that last bridge, they were in the country Caesar marched into two thousand years ago—to pacify (to rape and slaughter) what he named Gaul. Here, not ten years ago, the grand descendants of those Germanic tribes who overwhelmed Caesar's grand descendants pacified (raped and slaughtered) Gaul anew. Rape and slaughter, and peace. These strains cracked the voices of the lilies and the poppies of these meadows, their echoes resounding over the valleys as if the Great War's battles, and the Gallic Wars of aeons past, were being fought here this very twilight.

Yet, it was beautiful here, too, peaceful in the Gallic spring, the clime gentle, the earth awakening after her wintry slumber. After another week of travel, the caravan settled into the rolling hills of Provence to enjoy a long encampment, in what seemed a place finally free of marauding pursuers, a long awaited oasis in their forty years of wandering. The Spanish gadjo who had pursued them these long years were hundreds of miles south, on a peninsula where they, the Hebrews, were no longer. The mountain range was their Nile, Theo and Guaril laughed peacefully over those spring days, and Pharaoh's men were drowned there in some Andorran hot spring like in that Cecil B. Demille flick they'd gone to for a laugh before they'd all left Paris.

Things were pleasant as March drifted to its end in the meadows of Provence. But just as they were settling in, and beginning for the first time in forever to feel a measure of peace, a group of gadjo purifiers, these gendarmes of the French Republic, came out of the darkness one night in early April and surrounded the camp. They searched the wagons, shouted and jostled the men, women, and children, and began to make arrests. Most all the Gitanos surrendered without a fight, knowing well this dance, having suffered its steps many times before. But Guaril grabbed a red-hot iron from the fire, and clobbered a copper right across the face, wounding him badly. Three other gendarmes grabbed the iron away and held him, cursing his black ass for daring to strike back. A sergeant put his pistol up to Guaril's temple, Theo crying curses and pleas for mercy, writhing in the arms of the two burly gendarmes who held him.

"**NO!**" he screamed.

Guaril did not writhe, did not beg. His eyes fixed on the moon.

The sergeant made his pretty Gallic tongue ugly, growling at the black boy, and squeezed his trigger.

A pound of the flesh in Guaril's skull exploded onto the vernal soil.

Chapter 14

Katharina was a person without a name. This is what she concluded, one afternoon in 1927, in the pale and deathly light of the hydrotherapy chamber. She'd been in the wet pack for longer than she could recall, and the sheets round her had long gone hot, shrunk tight round her body. She was suspended in the air, some feet from the bath where she'd been soaked in the freezing water with its needly jets, without the ability to move anything besides her fingers and toes. Her face was the only thing that was not wrapped in the sheets, and all she could see was the ceiling and the ropes fastened to it. She felt the moist and vile evidence of her own piss and shit, wound up tight to her body in the sheets. She did not know how long it had been—hours? days? All she wanted to do now was die.

This was actually a rare moment for her; she was *awake*. She did not really remember being awake for a long time, and she wondered then whether she was not, in fact, dreaming all this. Memories swam in her mind, swirling and spiralling, all in a detached way she did not really own. She wondered whether to pay attention to them, but without them, there would be absolutely nothing to think about. And, too, she figured, even in her semi-delirium, that somehow these fleeting memories, spinning round her mind (which was dead) were her only real aspects of identity. This was why she was a person without a name any more, because she could not really recall it. And she debated with herself whether she should any more bother making the effort to claim those shards of memory, whether she should fight any more.

Why not? she concluded. What else was there to do? If she did not think, she would feel, and paralysed in the hot sheets, in pain from not having moved in days, and disgusted with the faeces and all the rest of it, she decided to fight, at least once more, to remember.

She had been here for a long time, not just suspended from the ceiling in the hydrotherapy room (for that, she thought, was only a day or two), but in this *place*. A hospital. A sanatorium. A place where she might be "cured."

What was wrong with her? She recalled this. There was something about a melancholic condition, one that had plagued her most all of her life, even from childhood. This was a feeling rather than a memory, for she could not really recall her childhood. But she knew somehow that she had been melancholic, in the world outside this Hell.

But that was not the only thing she was to be "cured" of. These "doctors," these quacks, knew nothing of Magnus Hirschfeld or Iwan Bloch or any of the sexologists she'd read and quoted liberally, in between actualizing their ideas in the best language she knew—the language of her body, bound and beaten, sweaty and screaming. These quacks called her a person suffering from "nymphomania"—an actual pathology, a "disease" to them. This, she thought with a cough of a chuckle, she would never deny being "afflicted" with. She recalled being proud of it at one time. But, these people here, they did not want her pride. They wanted her— *what?*

To be cured. But that wasn't really it, either. Even if all this could cure her, it did not seem geared to do such. No. She was not going to be discharged from this hospital. That wasn't why she was here. Rather, she was here because they did not ever want to let her out. She was a prisoner, a hostage. Yet, worse. For prisoners are held for a sentence, a definite unit of time. Hostages are held for a ransom, which, once paid, allows them to go free. No. Katharina was to be held here until the world ended.

So, why not hasten that? Why not die? Surely they *would* kill her eventually, with all these "treatments." She did not believe in God, and she would not pray to Him. But, if she were to do so, she would pray they'd fuck up and drown her, as they'd almost done so many times before. Or, when they gave her those injections, and she slept for days and even weeks, to the point where the seasons outside her window changed like passing afternoons, with no memory, not even dreams, to mark the time—she hoped against hope that one season, she would not wake up.

She could not understand it. Yet, it all had to do with the narrative she sensed in those swirls, that which she'd once defined as her personality. Power. She hated it. She *knew* that. For, if it exists at all, it exists like this. So, damn its existence. That much she could still recall.

When she first got here, back—how long had it been?— never mind—that was too depressing to think about—when she first got here, it had been winter. Snow had been falling. She saw it, surreally beautiful on the grounds and gardens outside her barred mesh-glass window. Now, it was summer, high summer; she could tell the few times she could look out a window, and she heard birds chirping early, and the sun came early, and did not disappear again till late. It was not the first summer she'd spent here; and at least one time, turning over in her sleep, she'd noticed changing leaves outside, and snow again, and spring's lemon sunlight. When she first got here, she'd met with doctors, who explained to her that she was insane. Indeed, she did act like a maniac then. She cursed and writhed, in that straitjacket they kept her in for fully two weeks. But, that had passed. Something to do with the injections, and the pills they force-fed her. That had blotted out spring. And then, the deep-sleep therapy. Summer had come, without much fanfare, then autumn, winter, spring again, and now summer once more. She'd been sleeping most of the time.

Katharina, she told herself. Then, she smiled. *Katya.* That, too, had been a name. She still remembered that, in defiance of all of it. Yes. She'd had lovers, lovers who had called her that.

Where were those sweet boys now? They could be dead. And, doubtlessly, they must think *her* dead, by now. And, they would not be far wrong.

She felt herself yielding. She was being tortured, as she always knew the authorities—whichever their justification, whichever class or state or particular economic system of their cruelty—*Authority*, always—would torture her someday. But, these authorities, these tormentors, they were quite insane. For there was nothing that they wanted from her, but her suffering. They did not want information, or confession, or denouncing her comrades, or her simple terror at their power. No. They actually thought they were *curing her* somehow.

Or, at least, that must be what they thought. Because otherwise, they were just torturing her to torture her. Maybe she was being experimented on. Yeah, that could be it. She was a lab rat. And they wanted to know how much she would take before she just died.

At that moment, she wanted death. But, they wouldn't let her have that, either. Cruelty had led to something without a name. What name could she give it? Simple sadism, or hatred, was not enough to explain this. Capitalism, Communism, Fascism—these words didn't cover the reality of this. No. It had no name. No name, but Madness.

And, she, too, had no name. For, she had to make an effort to remember it. Now, just now, she'd forgotten again. Maybe she'd remember later. Oh well.

Maybe she should scream again . . .

Chapter 15

Theodor found himself in prison. There had been a trial, or some such functional formality, but he'd hardly paid any attention to that. The other Gitanos were either with him in the dock, deported, or disappeared. He'd not known their language more than the most paltry phrases, and could not speak with them. The authorities realized that he was not a Rom; but he was found living among them, and that was enough to convict him of vagabondage, of vagrancy—an unpardonable crime in a settled land. He was convicted of that, and violence against the Gendarmerie Nationale, and sent to a prison in Lyon for a sentence of three years.

He was lucky, he realized. This was France. It might have been Devil's Island. But, no. His God was merciful. As merciful as God ever was.

Guaril was dead. And his murderers were not sent to prison. No, they probably got a medal for it, or a promotion, or whatever rewards they gave to filthy pigs the world over. Every trace of him was burned to ash and dust—his body, his few clothes and possessions, his diary and his portfolio of years' worth of sketches and collages—all burned in the same fire he'd taken that red-hot iron from, and dealt his last blow of defiance of the racist world. The gendarmes burned everything of that camp they could, and impounded the rest. Nothing had survived, no history to be recorded. Theodor was in a daze for months. Alone, in a cloud. Then, as this passed, he found himself weeping.

The other prisoners spoke French, mostly, as did the warders, and Theodor after a time knew a few words, enough to get by. But he consciously refrained from really getting to know the tongue of his captors. He wasn't interested. He wasn't interested in that, or in anything else of life. He contemplated suicide. And, short of that, he deliberately got into fights with prisoners bigger than he, or guards, hoping they'd beat him or shoot him or some other way deliver him from this misery. He was not thinking about the great struggle of the working class any more. This prison was but a mirror reflection, a microcosm, of the prison that governments round the world were making of the whole civilisation outside. It was hopeless, now. He should never have left Berlin, he thought. He should have stayed there, made his stand, and died.

But, he hadn't stayed. He'd embarked on a journey which had delivered his two best friends to their deaths. He was alone, now. All the people he'd ever loved in his life had died, been lost, or betrayed him. He found himself starved on mouldy bread and brackish water in the dark holes of solitary, or beaten senseless and left for dead, or raped by ugly men who hated him, for his being German, for his being an anarchist, for his being just that guy over there who was alone. He'd ceased to fight it.

It was all part of it, and laughing cynically, hopelessly, the only way he ever laughed, the thing that came out of him when he really went into despair, and sobbing or staring silently lost its use—laughing, he almost welcomed all this torture. After all, he was alone. If he was on the outside, he'd still be alone. So, this place, this time, just ended up suiting his mood.

He began, in the depths of his solitary confinement, shivering from the cold, shitting in little piles on the floor, watching the rats and roaches get into it, then get into *him*—he began to crave his old company, to revisit his old loves. He heard them, talking to him, comfortingly sometimes, sometimes in sharpest accusation. He heard Guaril, telling him to be strong one minute, then cursing him for abandoning him the next. He heard Katya whispering her torments from somewhere beyond the earth, some heaven or hell where she was a prisoner, a prisoner just like him. And he heard his father, telling him that he'd done this all to himself, that he'd chosen—*hadn't he?*—the path that led him here.

This last voice was the worst. For in all Theodor could see, hear, taste, touch, there was a bit of his father's disappointment in it. He could have been so great, his father told him. But no, he'd chosen for himself the path of dishonour and disgrace. He hated Germany; yet now, he represented Germany, the object of all the hatreds that hadn't been soothed by the passing of the war, by the treaty, by the inflation that had made of his nation a race of paupers. He hated God; yet, he prayed to Him, to Her, to It, to Them—begging for the release of death. But then, he would have to spend eternity with It, or with the Devil, or all alone as he was now. Things could never be good again.

Theodor got sick. He came down with something the prison doctors said was TB. It wouldn't kill him, they told him, he straining to understand their French diagnoses. No. It wouldn't kill him, not for a while yet. But, he'd never, ever be the same.

Was this a gift of God? Was this what Theo had prayed for?

Perhaps it was.

And he laughed again.

Theodor was released from Montluc prison in August of 1929, and was promptly deported back to old Deutschland. By now, the voices of his past were dogging him far more viciously than the Communists or the Nazis ever could. He was never really free of them. But he kept that to himself. One thing he didn't want was to go to a madhouse. A madhouse was worse than a prison. In a prison, they fucked with your body. In a madhouse, they fucked with your soul. He knew enough about that to know that he would easily jump into a river, or slash himself up with a broken beer bottle, or pick a fight with a dozen Brownshirts, before he'd ever let himself be carted away to there.

He wandered across Germany, seeing the waste, the abyss it was being plunged into. The Nazis were doing well. The workers were still following the Communists. The Weimar government was swamped with problems of renewed inflation and unrest. It was all he could do not to do the things he thought of. For his father did not want him to die, and when he came close to ending it, the broken bottle jagged in his hand, his father was all comfort then, talking about Workers' Heaven, a great beer hall in the sky, and how he was happy. The voices did not want him to kill himself. For then they, too, would die.

Theodor got to Berlin by the end of 1929, having wandered about for some six months, hearing lies and truths and myths breathed by countless souls along the way, news of Deutschland and legends, impossibly old and impossibly new, watching the seasons pass from a mild, wet autumn to a cold and unforgiving winter. He walked the streets for days and nights, sleeping in alleyways, taking alms from passers-by, finding scraps of food in dustbins. He looked a mess. His face was scraggle and dirt, his eyes fierce and frightening. His clothes were rags upon a bony frame. He found a little solace in drinking, sharing bottles of flat beer or rancid wine with old men and young, who, moved to charity, told him about the coming rise of the country, armless, legless veterans, with swastikas or spears or sickles on the flags of their wheelchairs, their tricycles, on their hats, their arms, plastered across their chests. Yes, they said. Deutschland was about to change. This misery could not go on forever.

They must have seen something in Theodor, something of the misery they all sensed around them, personified in his little body, in the insanity of his eyes. They, too, were crazy. And they had a respect for his greater madness, as if they had not the courage to go as far out as he. At least, this was how Theodor judged it.

He was sharing a bottle of stolen gin with an old, gammy-legged sailor on New Year's Eve, listening dumbly as he talked of mutiny, then fondly, wistfully of the Kaiser, in the park where he once made love to Katya—were they sitting on the very same bench?—and laughing sadly at the old man's jokes, listening without comment as the man mocked Nazis, Jews, queers, and police by turns, when he saw something that filled him with a feeling so strange he didn't really know what it was. He'd felt it before, in a deep, misty past, and he concentrated, to realize it was happiness. For the first time in a thousand years, he saw a face that was familiar.

"Johanna!" he croaked out to the figure, walking amidst the shanties. The figure stopped at the sound of the name. It came closer, moving out of the shadows. A woman stood before Theodor, a tall, pale, thickly beautiful woman, with long black hair beneath a huntsman's cap, the black and red gear of a nineteenth-century horsewoman, tight velvet trousers tucking into boots of poisonous green.

She squinted at him.

"No," she said to herself, but loud enough for him to hear.

"Johanna?" he squeaked again.

"No, it—it *can't* be—*Th-e-o?*"

Theo jumped to his feet and embraced her, more passionately than he'd ever have thought to embrace her in that past time, that murk of years ago, when he was happy. Though she hated men, more now than ever, the dark-haired beauty took him in her arms, and held him close.

"Jesu Maria, Theo!" she laughed in wonder and disbelief— "I thought you were dead!"

"I *am* dead," he said hollowly, his eyes moistening, his breath aflutter.

"Now, now. Come with me. You need a bath—and it seems like a hot meal wouldn't be a bad idea, either."

Johanna took him by the hand, and bade him be silent until they could get out of the park. They walked quickly, down the streets, down the alleys, to a tram which she paid for. She stared at him the whole time they were on the trolley, holding onto the wall since the straps to hang onto had all long been stolen, staring at him as if he were a ghost. He stared back. She had changed. It seemed she'd aged a good ten or twenty years since he'd last seen her, thinner, greyer, her face wrinkling and her eyes joyless. And, of course, he'd not aged any better. They kept looking at each other as if they weren't really sure they were dreaming. At length, they got off the tram, going into a pretty and subdued neighbourhood on the West End, where she was still living, apparently.

Johanna had money. She'd socked a lot away over the last five years, and still saw clients, though not so much for straight sex any more. She still wielded her whips and riding crops with alacrity, and catered to the darker tastes of the men of Berlin. They evidently still had an appetite for such things, and she was happy to oblige.

The place Johanna stayed in was a whole floor of a building, divided into smaller apartments, and managed by an old lady who maintained a laissez-faire attitude toward her boarder. There were many people living here, but Johanna really didn't speak to any of them. Her trade, after all, was not embraced by most people, the un-hep stupid people, of which Berlin still had more than its share. Yet, she was the richest among them, and people left her alone. She paid her rent six months in advance, so when they entered the house, the old proprietress smiled kindly to her and offered her some tea.

"Yes, Frau Essen," she said gaily, "that'd be lovely."

"I'll bring it to you right away, Fraulein Snyder," the old woman said, as if she were her servant, "right away," and she regarded Theodor with a courteous detachment, obviously figuring him for a client. Johanna opened a sliding door, and led him into her chambers.

"She seems friendly," Theo remarked, feeling like himself again, not really recognizing the feeling, it had been so long. Johanna, too, was returning to herself, the self he remembered, saying sharply, "She oughtta be—I'm the only one here who pays her anything like the rent on time."

Theo collapsed in an armchair instantly, his legs giving out as he laughed hollowly, incredulously.

He was home again!

Chapter 16

Johanna realized her old friend was far gone, and though she wondered where he'd been these last years, she didn't press him. She let him stay with her for several days and nights, in which time he washed, ate, and slept. He slept for almost twenty-four hours the first night, not waking till the end of the next day. Finally, he began to get himself to himself once again, and reflected on his past years, a long, twilit blur. After a few days and nights, he found himself talking to her, sharing with her, catching up.

He told her about Guaril. He told her about prison. He told her about despair, and even the voices which were even now rattling the windowpanes with the winter wind. To all this, Johanna just shook her head a little, and looked on in sympathy. She told him about herself. Things were not so good with her, either. She'd been diagnosed with syphilis. It was running its course through her body, and it was making her a little crazy, too. She knew it would only be a matter of time before she'd die of it, and she vowed to end it before she was shipped away to some charity sanatorium, to waste away in the final stages of dementia as the new law would allow any bastard health inspector to send her at his arbitrary, bureaucratic whim. Theo told her of his TB. They looked at each other a moment; then, they just laughed.

"Life's such a joke," she chuckled, "ain't it, Theo?"

"Yeah, it is," Theo laughed. "What the hell should we do?"

"What can we do?"

The question unanswered, they talked on. One thing she told him that brightened the horizon was that she knew for a fact that Katya was not dead. She'd been committed to a mental asylum, and she even knew which one. She'd been kind of waiting for her to get released. Just waiting. She was very close to Katya, and had not really been happy since she'd left Berlin. She'd received a letter from her, and that's how she knew she was still alive. Alive, but not well. The letter had none of the flair and style that had characterized Katya. It was almost illegible, a scrawl that looked and read like that of a six-year-old. It basically just said where she was, and not to worry, and that she was perfectly happy to spend her time there until she was "cured."

"That doesn't sound like Katya," Theo said.

"No," Johanna said. "No. They must have her on some horrid drugs. I tried to visit her, but they wouldn't let me in. That was about a year and a half ago. I thought, I'd love to do something, but . . . what can I do?"

"Can I see the letter?"

Johanna looked at him with a bitter amusement.

"Sure, I suppose," she said, as if it were a rather ridiculous request. Theo did not react to this. When he got the letter in his hands, though, he did react. He read between the lines scrawled in dark blue ink upon the light blue stationery, with the hospital crest embossed above it, and a postscript from some doctor informing whomever was intended to be the reader that the letter was "approved." Evidently, the quack didn't realize it would go beyond the ward. It was nothing but a memo to another doctor, as if the writing were an exercise. Suddenly, the full force of the thing struck Theo, deep and to the heart. They'd made her like this. And they were so arrogant that they didn't even understand that somebody else would read it. Evidently, they'd put it in the post thinking it would never be delivered. "My friend," as the salutation read, and the letter was addressed, must have been considered a figment of Katya's imagination.

"Fuck this," Theo said, softly, hotly. Then, he looked up at Johanna, and said, "We gotta get 'er outta there."

"I'd love to, liebschin," Johanna said, her voice a resigned sigh, "but how?"

"This is criminal. There's nothing wrong with Katya."

Johanna raised her brow, and almost laughed.

"*Now* there is," she said. "Just *look* at that, Theo. If she wasn't crazy when she got there, she sure is crazy now!"

Theo shook his head.

"No," he said. "She might be drugged, fucked up—but she's still her! You gotta understand, sister, I've been in a fog for four years and more, thinking she was dead. So, she's in a fog, too. So what? She *ain't* dead! She's just wasting away in that place, rotting there. She probably thinks we're *all* dead! If thinking that could fuck *me* up, and they weren't even putting me on drugs and brainwashing me—what would it be like for her?"

"What's your point?"

"My point is that she can come back! Just like I'm beginning to. All she needs is to be around the people she loves again."

"Okay, Theo. Sure. But *how* do we get her out? She's evidently been certified as insane. Once some quack doctor does that, they can keep her there indefinitely, as long as they say she's insane. Evidently, her family's paid some quack off, to certify her as mad. What are we gonna do, Theo?"

"I'll *break* her outta there, if I have to!"

"Oh, sure. Just like that commie Olga Benario busted out her lover from the prison in the Mitte last year, right? That's very romantic, Theo—*but it can't work.*"

"Why not? They never caught her or Li De, did they? I heard about it when I was on the road—before I even got to Berlin. The commie bums couldn't talk enough about it."

"No, they didn't catch them, Theo. But they had a place to run to. D'you think you could find asylum in Russia, you and Katya? Like those two famous Communist Party members? You'd end up in a *Russian* prison, then, some Gulag! There's no country for us, Theo, no motherland. We've just got the fucking Fatherland. You try to get her out that way, and you'll be locked up again—*both of you*—or you'll be on the run for the rest o' your naturals! We've got nothin', man. Face it. We've got nothing we can fight with."

A thought occurred to Theo.

"She was to get an inheritance," he remembered. "Almost a hundred million marks—pre-war value—in gold. From her great aunt in Switzerland. If we can prove that her parents put her there, just to rob her of her inheritance—I mean, shit! That's a case!"

Johanna considered.

"Yeah, it is," she said finally. "Yeah, Theo, it is. . . . I've actually a couple clients who are lawyers. I suppose I could get one of 'em to file charges against her parents, or the hospital, or something. Yeah, I could. I mean, if she's been wrongly fucked out of her inheritance, and we could say that, well . . . all we'd need is a psychiatrist to contest the diagnosis. *That* could be hard."

Before Theo could comment, Johanna was smiling, evilly, very sure of herself once again. She looked twenty years younger in that moment.

"No, it won't be!" she corrected herself. "There's a helluva lotta psychiatrists we can get—hell! If those bastards can buy one—so can we! And it'd be easier, probably, for us, because we don't hafta get the shrink to lie. I've some cash saved up, Theo. I could get a little bribe together. . . . Of course, I'd be vulnerable. If the Von Rosen family was out to get us, it'd be pretty easy to fuck me up. My chosen trade, 'n' all, and the new law—my forged *Gesundheitszeugnisse*—I still won't register with those pricks—

damn 'em to hell! All that, *all* that darling . . ."

"I'll make the bribe," Theo decided. "You give me the money, and I'll get the shrink. You won't be traced. That family doesn't know any of us well. I mean, they probably have spies, just like any other high-up capitalist bastards—but, you stay the fuck away from it. I'll take all the risks. Hell! It's not like I don't know what prison is. Not like it scares me any more"

"There *is* something else they can do to you, Theo, you know."

"Johanna, I love Katya. So do you. Up till twenty minutes ago, I thought she was dead. And the way it is now, it's almost like she *is* dead. Almost like *I'm* dead. So what? They get some thugs to beat me up? Or kill me? It's not like we're not dyin' anyway!"

Johanna chuckled.

"That's true," she said. "Okay, Theo. Sure. I'll talk to my lawyer friends. And you find some psychiatrist that'll contest the certification. I'll give you a thousand marks right now—it's a mix of Rentenmarks and Reichsmarks, more of the first than the second, I'm afraid—but I've got it. Just let me get it from my piggy bank, right here, behind these books. . . . When d'you wanna start all this?"

Theo took the wad of money she handed him, and stuffed it into the lining of his jacket. He looked out into the dawn.

"Right now," he said, softly, but with more confidence than he'd had in years.

He went directly out into the cold January dawn, his heart afire. He headed straight for the West End shopping district, and bought himself a set of posh clothes, the most expensive he'd ever dared buy. Looking curiously unlike himself, he prepared to make the connections he would need to make. He could walk the streets now without fear, no fear of Bullen, no fear of Brownshirts or Reds. He didn't look like himself any more.

He spent the next days getting appointments with psychiatrists, inquiring as if he were a slightly neurotic patient with a lot of cash what their specialities were, what theories they followed, how they viewed the subject of involuntary incarceration. Freudians he ruled out outright. Jungians and Adlerians he was more curious about, though feeling a few of them out, he concluded they weren't quite right, either. Finally, he got a younger fellow, who spoke highly of the sexual liberation theories of both Wilhelm Reich and Magnus Hirschfeld, erring when pressed toward the latter, and realized he'd struck gold.

Coyly, Theodor played out his little scenario, stating that he was interested in the theories of the geniuses he'd heard so much about, and that a certain friend of his had told him all he knew of these men. This, of course, was Katya. But, things had been hard for his friend, Theodor said, and he mentioned that she'd been improperly diagnosed in his opinion, by some Freudians.

"Yes," said the young man, eager-faced, blonde, bespectacled and almost boyish (though he was no younger than Theodor himself), "those fellows are a little slanted, I feel. . . . You're saying the fraulein you know has been *committed?*"

"Yes, Herr Doctor. All because the family did not approve of her . . . her 'lifestyle.' And most of that was because she was openly sexual—I mean to say, she was sexually liberated. . . . So . . . would you . . . would you agree to see her? And make your own evaluation?"

The fellow looked a little pained.

"I really don't know," he said. "Though I sympathize with you, Herr Priser, I'm really not that experienced. I'm just starting a practice here. Something like this could, well, it could *jeopardize* my future."

Theodor breathed.

"Herr Doctor, there are other aspects to this case. . . . See, the fraulein in question comes from a rather wealthy family. She stood to inherit a large sum of money from a departed relative, outside her immediate family. I feel—and I'm not alone in this— that she has actually been falsely committed, in order to prevent her from—from attaining her rightful fortune."

This admission, this letting of the young analyst into Theodor's confidence, was calculated. He was putting his cards on the table, not all of them, but enough. But Theodor miscalculated. The idea of legal complications only served to nonplus the doctor further. He got that pained look again, and was about to say something, when Theo decided to lay one last card down.

"Please, Herr Doctor, just see her. You're under no obligation. I mean, in the case. You are an impartial observer— that's all I want. And, if there was any matter of a retainer, for the privilege of your services, I would be more than happy to advance it. Right now. Without any obligation on your part."

"I don't know, Herr Priser. It's not really, I think, entirely ethical, to—"

"—Herr Doctor, this woman is my closest friend. I love her. I spent years thinking she was dead. She's been fit up, in my opinion, for the 'crime' of nymphomania—a disease you've already said you feel doesn't even exist. Can a future be ruined for that? A whole life, forfeit, because of the backwardness and guile of unethical men who use your profession, not for healing, but for its opposite? I'm not *bribing* you, Herr Doctor! I'm *begging* you, for common human decency's sake, and for the integrity of your profession, to be—to be *fair* to her—and to give her the chance to clear herself from a label which you *know* is nothing but sexism and repression! I mean, Herr Doctor—think about it! You could make a name for yourself—with one act—an act of kindness, an act of charity—but more, an act which would prove to the world the worth of psychiatry, and the goodness of sexuality and freedom, as Reich, Hirschfeld, Bloch, Eulenburg—and *you yourself* defend."

Theo had more cards in his hand than he'd figured. He came in here to make a bribe. He'd played that hand. But, now, he was impassioned, telling it exactly as it was. There was no more guile on his part. He was giving this man in all honesty the direction he knew he would value. As he regarded the young doctor's face, looking down, timidly, but with a glimmer of possibility, Theo got up.

"I'm sorry to take up your time, Herr Doctor," he said coldly. "If you can't do this, I understand. Maybe, though, you could recommend someone who I could speak to next? I don't care how many people I have to talk to—there *must* be someone who follows new thoughts in the profession who would be open to evaluating my friend. Someone with the courage to follow through with their enlightened theories. I think—"

"—No, Herr Priser," the young man said, looking up, "no, that won't be necessary. You're quite right. There's no shirking this. It's a responsibility. I'll do it. And, I'll require no *retainer—* beyond my usual fee."

Theodor smiled, and shook the young doctor's hand.

"Thank you," he said. "You're a credit to your profession—whatever your diagnosis is."

The man regarded him with a slight embarrassment. He'd been shamed into this. But, shame, though his training went against the principle, had efficacy in his case. He was, he knew, staking his reputation on the line. He would have to take on the Establishment, for he knew even before he'd met Katya that she was not insane.

That people were chucked into asylums unfairly and without justification was no revelation to this man. And he forgave Theodor for his almost-insult, because he realized the fellow loved her, and desperately. Poor creature, the doctor thought, looking to Theodor. Here was a poor and uneducated fellow, who had bought a new suit, out-of-fashion and ill-fitting, who could not even open his mouth without revealing his lower class origins—though he tried—who must have fallen in love with a rich girl, and she with him—and for that "crime," she'd been sent away. Yes, the doctor thought, I shall do it—damn the consequences, the retaliations of any entrenched party. For my profession, for fairness, for this creature before me and his love, and, for *myself*—I shall see this through.

Theodor found he won his hand, the winning card something he had not intended to play; indeed, it was a card he never knew he had.

Chapter 17

Katharina awoke, finding herself in a wheelchair, being carted off for yet another treatment. What would it be this time? Hydrotherapy? The wet-pack? The spinning pendulum-chair? More drugs? She no longer cared.

Sighing, she closed her eyes, and did not open them again till she found herself in a room she had never been in in all the years she'd known this place. The Visitor's Room.

Visitors? In all her years here, Katharina had never had a visitor. She wondered if anyone in her life even cared about her any more, whether they even wanted to know her. She felt disgraced. She had lost control. She had given in. She no longer struggled when they force-fed her pills, no longer refused the slop they fed her, probably mixing up all kinds of hateful things into the mush. She did not smile; but she did not frown, either. Not now.

Who was visiting her?

She saw the further door open, as her attendants fell back, but did not leave. Three men walked in, along with a woman. They sat down on the other side of the table the attendants had pushed her to.

Katharina viewed them all as if she were having a dream, and not one she was likely to remember. It was hazy, as all things were hazy for her, and she recognized no one. They were just four people, whom she had no way of knowing were not just agents of the authorities here. More doctors, more quacks. This was probably yet another experiment. She was a lab rat . . .

Then, she heard her name.

"Katya?"

The man who said this said it in a voice that she'd reconciled herself to never hearing again. Katharina looked up, squinting in puzzlement, trying to place the face of the sandy-brown bearded man in the new suit.

Then, her eyes widened. The man's face—the *boy's* face— though old and careworn, alcoholic-wasted, crazy—this face was *her* face. It belonged to her, as did the person who wore it.

An experiment? Was this another mind game, in the endless series of mind games they'd played on her over the long years of this exile? Could this person be—

"—*Theo?*"

The face smiled, and all the years that pocked and wrinkled

it fell away.

"Yes, Katya," he said, reaching over his hand across the table. She instantly took it.

"Oh, God!" she cried—"My God! Theo! And—and—Johanna—*darling!*"

Johanna put her hand across the table, and the three joined hands in a touch more passionate than lovemaking. They felt each other's hands, and Katya reached down and kissed them both. They wanted to embrace, to cry, to laugh, to celebrate! But the attendants were still there behind Katharina, and were making sure that this contact would be the only one they had.

Katya could not believe what was happening. She must be dreaming—she must be! But for the first time in forever, the dream was *good.* She'd recall it fondly the next time they put her in the wet-pack, and she was left with her memories, her only companions in Hell.

"We're *real*, darling," Johanna said, anticipating her thoughts, reading her glazed expression. "We're here for you—at last."

"Can you please stick to the agenda of your business," came a voice behind Katya. To this, one of the unfamiliar men, the elder of the two, pulled out a paper from his briefcase, and said, just as coldly, that his "client" and he had things to discuss, and it was illegal for these orderlies to molest him in his business.

"If you'd kindly leave us alone," he said curtly, "I think we can proceed."

The attendants stared at this man, almost bemused.

"Please," said the man, though his tone was commanding, not beseeching, "please gentlemen, don't make me have to file a report to the government. Kindly leave us in peace."

The hospital functionaries realized from his bearing and manner that this was a man of power, as powerful as they were, if not more so. They waited a moment more, while the lawyer stared at them, then one of them contented himself by limiting their time to fifteen minutes. This was agreed upon, and the hospital staff left them all there, alone.

With the staff gone, Theo and Johanna shot up and embraced Katya with all the affection she'd been starved of these last four-and-a-half-years. Katya was slow, disbelieving, effects of the brainwashing they'd done to her for longer than she could remember. But she hugged them back, a glimmer of feeling breaking through the haze.

"I—" she stammered—"I thought—you were dead—both of you."

"We thought you were, too," said Theo. "But, you're *not dead*, Katya. You're gonna be released from this awful place. These men are Herr Roth and Herr Lieber. They're a lawyer and a doctor, respectively. Doctor Lieber here is going to evaluate you, for the purpose of determining your—your competency."

"And Herr Roth," explained Johanna, "is a personal friend of mine, who has agreed to take your legal case."

"My what?"

"Your case, Fraulein Von Rosen," Herr Roth said. "There are grounds for action, against the parties which put you here. You have a sum of money to which you've been denied."

Katya looked up at him.

"Yes," she said absently, just coming into her own, "yes, my inheritance. Yes."

"Precisely, Fraulein Von Rosen. It is our contention that you've been falsely held here, these past several years. Though, even if that cannot be proved, we can make a case for your release, pending Doctor Lieber's examination, and then attend to the matter of suing your family for the estate you were ruled not competent then to inherit."

Katya shook her head. Like a wave of orgasm, a great surge of feeling came over her, washing up over her body and brain, threatening to drown her in joy. Yes! She was who she was! They hadn't stolen it from her, after all!

Over the next days, Dr. Lieber conducted his evaluation. The patient was slow, performing poorly on a standard IQ test, at least compared with the high scores she'd had when originally tested, some ten years before. But that, in itself, did not speak against her competency. Dr. Lieber knew well the reasons for the poor performance. This patient had been subjected to mind-altering, mind-damaging "treatments"—non-stop—for going on half a decade. Dr. Lieber was of a radical school in psychiatry; he felt most of the supposed treatments of the mentally ill were only designed to make things worse. But he was clever enough not to talk about this. He confined himself to strict empirical evidence, test scores, universally acknowledged, which proved the patient was no threat to herself or others. There was no reason to keep her in this dungeon any more.

Herr Roth's firm filed suit against the Von Rosens, and there were some machinations back and forth between his firm and the several retainers the Von Rosen shipping line had working for it. Legal dances were danced, appeals, counter-appeals, injunctions, more appeals—till somebody upstairs in the Von Rosen offices finally understood the firm of Herr Roth could neither be bought off nor bullied. With liberal use of a press hungry for sensationalism, intrigue, corruption, anti-capitalism and anti-Semitism, the holdings of the great conglomerate of companies was finally forced to the table. The ensuing trial proceeded over the next months, over the late spring and early summer of 1930. Witnesses from both sides debated and testified. Court-appointed experts were called in, as supposedly neutral arbiters. But the chicanery of courts, bribes, and untoward expertise was not enough to prejudice the case. For money has one sure enemy, and that's more money. Katya promised half her inheritance to the lawyers who could set her free. And Herr Roth and his firm proved sharp and capable agents of Weimar law. It was eventually ruled a gross miscarriage of justice, Katharina Von Rosen's false imprisonment for nearly five years in a sanatorium whose main underwriters were the girl's scheming family. In the bad press against the Von Rosen family, who were after all Jewish bourgeois in a time and place that frowned on that, public opinion was such that it seemed a little telling, and more than a little rotten, to pervert psychiatry to disinherit a wayward daughter of her rightful fortune.

Of course, Katya came to laugh, it was sneaky, in a way, to bring out the dirty laundry of her family, in a climate that was so hungry for such dirty laundry. And, too, what good were courts and laws, anyway, to a woman who hated both? A poor person would have been lost in the bedlams of the state, never to be heard from again. But Katharina would soon be a person of property, and that made all the difference.

The press had a field day with the story. The Nazis called it evidence of Jewish corruption. The Communists called it evidence of bourgeois decadence. The Catholic Centrists bewailed the loss of God. Everybody had their own spin on it. And with the money Johanna was fronting, and the favours she was calling up, as well as (in small part, to be sure) the actual injustice of the case, it all served Katya well. The Von Rosen shipping line began to lose contracts, and the government began to bear down hard on the now hated family. Katya was awarded her release, and soon thereafter most of the fortune—gold equivalent to billions and billions of Papiermarks nowadays, quite more than a few million Reichsmarks—that were her due.

The victorious daughter would never speak to her parents again, and she gave away a lot of her money, rewarding various causes (including Herr Roth's firm) for their patience and commitment. Katya didn't even want the money any more. She just wanted to be left alone. And within a few months, nobody knew her any more. The brief notoriety of the case passed into the oblivion of a world with more pressing issues to contend with. Government scandals, elections, sensational *lustmord* sex-murders, and the deepening of the worldwide Depression following the crash of the stock market last year, served to return Katya to happy anonymity by the fall. The media had used her, the tide of anti-Semitism was just a little stronger in her country now, and she was effectively an orphan.

But, she was free.

Chapter 18

Life had long been surreal. For the past years, Katya and
Theo had dwelt in the netherworld, prison and the madhouse, taken
from the lives they once knew, which, though it had never been
pretty, was something they found themselves longing for like a
Paradise Lost. Sanity. Sometime, some place, there had been
sanity. But now, the hope for that world had spiralled off into
nonsense and oblivion, long, long lost, like some mythic, hoary
legend of a past which they accepted as theirs, but could not rightly
remember, so that even then, even in the memories of the time
before, there was a cloud of unreality. The Tiergarten, where they'd
first made love, where they'd walked with Guaril; the Spree, which
they'd seen flowing past all their Berlin lives, where Theodor's
father's ashes had floated, till they became one with its flow; all the
memories of Wittenberg Platz and Passauer and Anbacher streets,
the glitz of the Potsdamer Platz and the shadows of the Alex; the
hidden haunts of the Black Tie and a Blue Moon; life on the East
End and the West End and the waterfront of the Mitte; all the
experiences of Berlin from the present moment back through
earliest childhood, now seemed, if not lies, then a queer and
distorted mirror image of reality, something in a sideshow fun-
house. Nothing seemed real, in the past, or in the present—let alone
the future. Nothing to hang onto. Nothing, but each other.

Katya, moved by a need to find the thread of reality she
convinced herself must be there, somewhere, some bridge between
the myth of past and the insane anhedonia of the present, tried to
rent the very flat where she'd lived before all the madness began.
She found the landlord, a slum-lord of the Alex, and paid him a
year's rent in order to convince him to let the place to her.

Theo and Katya stood there, in the empty rooms, the walls
still the same faded brown floral, faded further than before, the
floors buckled now and bare. All her furniture, pictures, carpets,
books, everything long gone, long stolen by the tenants who had
come later. The door she'd paid extra to install there was replaced
by some flimsy thing, somebody recognizing the quality of the
wood and absconding with it outright, leaving the slum-lord to
kvetch about the filth he'd rented to throughout the 'twenties, who
had no morals of any discernible kind, who stole from him, who
failed to pay him even a month's rent. The old man was so happy to
rent to her, a "woman of quality," that he didn't think to ask any

questions about who she was, where she'd been, quite forgetting that she'd been his tenant herself years ago, one of the hundreds of nameless, faceless "filth" he'd been leaching off and cursing as long as he'd had the property. Katya said nothing. She just signed the lease, and the cheque, and moved in.

So now, here they were, in the empty parlour, looking to the sliding doors that had jumped their tracks, at the windows all filthy in the far room where she and Johanna had made love. Could you come home again?

They went through the rituals of love, there on an old mat on the floor, taking to them as poetry they'd loved and lain down in times of innocence that they struggled to make sense of now, reading it as in a foreign tongue they'd once mastered, but had fallen out of practice with till now they were hopelessly rusty. Their heads and hearts only half into it, they tried for a passion that had been so free and easy between them, once upon a time. As she lay back, Theo tasted her, felt her, endeavoured to please her. Her orgasm was so far away, and had been so long to her a stranger, she wondered now if she would ever feel it again. And she tasted him, felt him, told him coy and dirty stories she made up, slowly, slowly bringing them both back from the abyss. They did not know whether they'd come, neither Theo nor Katya; but there was solace in it.

"Well," she smiled in the first light of dawn, filtering in through windowpanes even filthier than they remembered, "here we are, Theo."

"Yeah. It feels and smells kinda the same."

Katya took a deep breath, savouring the scents of waxed wood and smoke and stale whiskey that she'd thought of as her own peculiar perfume, scents that had no meaning in themselves, but combined into something like comfort.

"We can find some furniture in the trash," she said, feeling suddenly almost gay, "just like before. And books . . . we need books, Theo. And a good cabinet to keep schnapps, and wine, and things."

"A bed might be nice, too," Theo chuckled as they lay on their buckled floor, remembering like a dream the great canopy bed that was big enough to sleep three people so comfortably, him, her, Guaril.

"Yeah," she said. "But what we really need are the people. Where are the people, Theo?"

Over the next days and nights, they tried to find people. Most had cleared out of Berlin, without trace. Many others had gone communist. A lot of the young people who in the early years were anarchically-inclined, had come to think of red as meaning the flag of that country to the east. They had clubs, bars, salons—crazy places, fun places, all the things the rathskeller they'd once loved as The Black Tie had had, that Mecca of anarchy long, long gone, piles of rubbish and scrap coal now filling that cellar in the dark. The Red establishments were vibrant, daring, the clothing queer, the music hot, the art wondrous, open late into the night. But, this was only because the commies had stolen what had been anarchist culture, allowed it to flower in all its bohemian splendour, but under a counterfeit sun, the nourishing rain blood from secret Gulags in far away Siberia. Few knew about those places yet. A younger generation had come up who thought a Red Revolution would deliver a nation of clubs and bars and salons, that this freedom would last forever. Even people like Kurt Weill and Berthold Brecht, who had written the soundtrack and subtext of much of what was radical in Berlin throughout the last decade, were now members of the KPD. Even former surrealists, those poets and poetesses who defied even anarchist conformities, had begun to be seduced by the hammer and sickle. Louis Aragon, that beautiful man who had so passionately condemned white civilisation in that talk in Madrid Katya and Theo had seen with Guaril the last summer they were together, had (they heard) become a card-carrying member of the French Communist Party in 1927, and had even written a poem praising its chairman. The commies were eating everything liberatory, and spitting it out again as skeletal caricatures, all saluting Moscow with the stiff arm of a Nazi Heil (so Theo phrased it bitterly). The cafés round town now were peopled with the denizens of cell meetings, armchair planners of strikes and demonstrations—either that or petty-bourgeois pseudo-intellectuals who liked debate for sophistry, and clung to communism as a means to be included in all the drama. None of these seemed to get what Katya and Theo meant when they said theory and life were not meant to be separate entities.

The new crowd was sometimes hopeful, sometimes cynical, all mixing into a rising, paranoid anxiety. The Depression made everyone think the malaise of the German economy would only worsen, and something drastic would have to be done, and soon. Lenin was long dead. Bukharin had been liquidated in a torturous show trial, and Trotsky had been driven out of Russia. A man named Stalin had emerged from the shadows, and was organizing the patronage machine in Russia, making adherence to its orthodoxy tighter and tighter amongst the Communist Parties abroad. The Communists here in Germany were doing better each election. So were the Nazis. Hitler was out of jail. You could hear him speak on the radio now, his thunderous voice like the ravings of a demented clown, Katya sneered. But nobody else was laughing. Her parents were clearing out, selling their assets, and moving to Palestine.

Theodor found nobody was following him any more. It had been more than five years since he'd written anything, and people had forgotten. That was just as well. He'd lost the will for politics.

Though they tried to mix into the new crowd, Katya and Theo found themselves ostracised for clinging to anarchy. Old friends turned a cold shoulder to them, or would argue for hours and hours and whole nights, citing strange, daft theories to prove what both Theo and Katya could refute with the ease of common sense. The forced collectivization of the farms in Russia, the liquidation of the kulaks, the suppression of all political dissent—these things required a "deeper understanding" the old friends said, required dialectics and a grasp of history. But Theo knew this game of dialectics, knew his history, and could laughingly perform the mental gymnastics necessary to "grasp" their old friends' new theories. He trounced the arguments till the old comrades turned away in disgust. Katya, for her part, turned from *them* in disgust, and banished them as surely as they banished her. It led them to feel very alone again, in a city that, more even than in the old days, seemed to be going mad.

So much had happened since they'd both been forced away from the world. The Italian anarchists in America, Sacco and Vanzetti, long a cause to fight for amidst all the rest of anarchist activism during the 'twenties, had been executed the year before last; and no uprising had followed in that capitalist cradle, the U.S.A., nor anywhere else to protest it. Severino Di Giovanni, who had answered the injustice with his own propaganda of the deed—bombings across several countries of newspapers and embassies and capitalist enterprises that had campaigned for and supported Sacco and Vanzetti's state-murder—had been caught and executed along with his comrades. His violence had divided what little remained of anarchist circles, here in Germany and all over the world. There were some who defended Di Giovanni, sympathizing with his actions, either for their desperation or for their bravery—or because what else could a concerned human being do in the wake of such cynical murder by the state, when mass movements to free Vanzetti and Sacco had come to nothing? What else could a person who valued freedom and justice do, if not *act* against the injustice? Yet there were many more anarchists who said Di Giovanni's actions served the powers that be—an excuse for outright military dictatorship in Argentina, where many of his targets had been. It left Katya and Theo and those few who were with them very confused, bemused. If mass action did not work, and individual direct action likewise was doomed—what, finally, could anyone do?

The situation round the world had soured on other fronts, too, during the years Theodor rotted in a French prison, and Katharina languished in a madhouse. One of the great revolutionaries from America, the I.W.W. anarcho-syndicalist "Big Bill" Haywood, had died of alcoholism in Russia in 1928. Rumours said after escaping life-imprisonment in America during the Red Scare of 1919 to come to Russia, finding asylum in the "Workers' Republic," he'd grown isolated and disillusioned in the nation he'd fled to. The Wobblies in America were almost dead, as all over the world—not just from repression by capitalist governments, but too, because of the defection of so many of their militant members to the Communist Parties. Communist seduction of anarchists and other revolutionaries was hatefully enticing; yet, the promised affair left many people despairing, and many more dead. An uprising of workers and students had taken over Shanghai, China in 1927, partially under Communist cadres' auspices. But bad advice from the Communist International, many said, had led to the uprising's isolation in the city, and a failure to spread the revolt elsewhere. The nationalists under Chang Kai-Shek had cut off the city, then, brutally putting down the rebellion, purging his own party of leftists of any stripe. Meanwhile, in Africa, the Riffian rebellion, which had seemed so strong in 1924 and 1925 against Spain and France when Katya and Theo and Guaril had been in those countries, had been entirely crushed by 1926. The cause of anti-colonial freedom had almost no champions left in Europe by the end of this turbulent decade. And all the wonderful men and women and even children who had tried to assassinate Mussolini, the Fascist leader of Italy, over their more than several attempts in the last years, had each failed to bring him down. A decade with hope was the 'twenties as it began, a decade whose turmoil promised great changes; but it was ending in defeat.

Katharina fell into a deep depression toward the last months of the year. As she slept in her new, second-hand twin bed through the shortening days and the long nights, Theodor sat at her feet, sipping cheap gin, having arguments with the world of hatreds in his head, which he heard rattling the windowpanes amidst the traffic noises and the rallies of the Hitler Youth burning radical books and books by Jewish writers of all kinds in the street below.

Then, on New Year's Eve, the last night of 1930, exactly a year after a broken Theodor had croaked out recognition for Johanna in the park, the beginning of life after so long a sojourn in limbo, Katya began to smile like she'd had so long ago, and told Theo that all this misery would not do.

"We're still alive, goddammit!" she declared, shouting it as loudly as the groans of the orgasms they'd finally begun to experience together again.

"So we are," Theo smiled softly. "So we are."

"It's New Year's Eve! The last official day of this miserable decade!" she laughed defiantly—"I'm gonna ring Johanna! And then the three of us'll do the town! Just like old times! That lesbian bar's still there, on the corner—*pretty, pretty old place . . .*"

"You know," Theo mused thoughtfully, "I've never actually been inside."

"Really? Oh, that's a *crime*, Theo—a *crime!* I'll ring Johanna, straight away, and we'll go there—this very night!"

Johanna had been drinking a sad, lonely fifth of vodka in her rooms in the West End in the dark, deciding to forgo the celebrations of yet another year older. She was just drifting into a dreamless reverie, on her way to stupor, when the phone sharply cut through her haze. She lifted the receiver to her ear and almost shouted at it.

"Well, then!" Katya laughed. "You'll be a cheap drunk tonight!"

"Who the hell—?"

"C'mon, girlfriend. You don't remember the best bottom you ever topped?"

"Oh . . . oh . . . Katharina."

"Very good, darling! Maybe you can tell me where you've disappeared to for the last five months, eh? I've been *craving* you,

you know."

"I've been . . . busy."

"Doing what?"

The voice over the phone rasped hard into Katya's ear.

"*Dying*, you stupid bitch! What *else?!*"

"Just like me, huh? Lemme tell you something. We're not going to heaven, Johanna. Either way, whether there is one or there isn't. D'you know that, m'girl?"

There was growling on the other end of the line. Finally, the growling took the form of words: "*Fuck Jesus! Fuck the Pope!—and fuck the Virgin Mary, too!!*"

Katya chuckled in triumph.

"Now *that's* the Johanna I remember! C'mon, suße, I don't hold your absence against you; I've been brain-dead and soul-starved over the last half year, too. But fuck it, man! You don't wanna just fade out, do you? Remember that Yank poetess, Edna St. Somebody-or-other? You used to quote her after you beat me till my backside was bloody. Something about a candle, lit at both ends??"

Johanna in her little tomb smiled wryly, thinking to Katya's bare, wide, beautiful dusky eggshell ass red and striped and glistening. Yes, that was a sight she liked to see.

"'It gives a lovely light,'" she murmured.

"Right! So, why don't you meet us at our little haunt, the place we met ten years ago tonight? Y'know, the place that changes its name every three months or so—every time they have to close down 'cause of the Bullen—then they reopen it again under a different name? Believe they're calling it 'Pandora's Box' lately—cute, huh?—after that Louise Brooks flick last year—*God!* That gal was *hot* in it! And *cool, beautiful*—the only truly good soul in a world of money-grubbing, filthy, *lustmord*-happy men! Saw the second run of it the weekend I was released from the nut-house. Made me wet for *months*—all those *icky* situations she got herself into! Put *myself* in them, y'know—blackmailed, compromised, sold into sex-slavery in Cairo—*immolated* at the end! Ah! Fun stuff!! 'Course, I *am* a sicko, am I not, darling? . . . You remember the night we met, *meine grausam Göttin?* when that place didn't even have a proper name yet? I'd been to half-a-dozen places, the Toppkeller Club, the Geisha, the Esplanade, the Domino-Bar—hell! I even went to that death-trap closet bar, the Eldorado, where all the straights go to gawk and blackmail people—looking for a woman who'd know how to be both femme *and* tough as hell—so rare, the woman who can be pretty and tough, too, liebling. Remember how I came in all bedraggled, my mascara running, my skirt ruffled—shameless slut I was! Remember how you threw your drink at me when I tried to buy you one? How you stuck my head in the water closet in front of all those pretty scorpions I'd been throwing myself at, and made me promise I'd get your name branded on my left asscheek?? Y'know, we never did do that, liebling. What say, you come out of retirement tonight, and we go over there and see if their fireplace still works? All those long, sharp fire-pokers, just collectin' dust . . ."

Johanna laughed till she giggled.

"All right, you sick horny little bitch," she spat in loving hate at her receiver. "You want some Jack-the-Ripper knife-play to end your seductress career, my little Pandora? Maybe I'll carve my initials into you, under the mistletoe—or maybe I'll leave a nice little cattle-brand on your sweet ass, so you remember me when I go."

And she hung up.

"Johanna's in?" Theo asked.

"Yes," Katya grinned, a private, anticipating grin. "But—wait a moment, liebling." She picked up the phone, dialled, and said: "Bring a change of clothes, would you, schätzele? No, not for you or me. . . . Yes, darling—something," Katya looked Theo up and down, "*skimpy . . .*"

The old dyke bar was not the friendliest place to Theo's kind, boys straight *or* boys gay—and the gals there had every reason to have this enmity. Straight boys were rapists and murderers, almost as often as they were creepy voyeurs and tourists come to colonize the gals' scene with their unwelcome leers and comments. And the gay boys nowadays were as often as not classist pricks, readers of *Der Eigenen—The Self-Owned*—glorying in privilege and looking down on the female-bodied hardly less than the Ancient Greek philosopher-pederasts they emulated. Pandora's Box was a shade less man-hating than the Monacle-Bar, maybe, where the big *Bubi* dykes were said to beat up men who flashed man-ness savagely just for *thinking* of entering, just for hanging round within a block of its doors. Maybe a shade less man-hating, Pandora's was—but *just.*

Theo, though, more than ever before, saw himself losing any allegiance to that old patriarch of a spirit that made him masculine. Not that Katya minded his masculinity; she adored him, for the strength of his arms, for the hot look of longing in his eyes, his taking her in some fairytale conquest she and he both gloried in. These flavours were among the ones they'd enjoyed rediscovering over these last months. But Katya wanted something different to mark this anniversary, something she and Johanna talked about many times in that lost era of before, something that had stirred Theo's profile into tumescence on hearing of their plans, but had never yet tried. Katya hinted in the next hour, but did not say outright. When Johanna arrived, stumbling elegantly through the old flat's threshold, tossing her empty vodka bottle shattering down the stairs, all was clear.

Theo smiled at the lingerie, the slutty seams running down grey hosiery stockings, the pretty patent-leather flats, the skirt he recognized as the same sexy, silky tassel-fringed miniskirt Katya had been wearing when he first met her, first kissed her in that alley nearly a decade ago, along with the same diaphanous, lacy top, and said to them both: "You know, I think I could fit quite nicely into those."

Katya and Johanna looked at him. Katya's face lit up, and Johanna's took on an old and sisterly satisfaction. "Yes, my little girlie boy," the latter said, in a voice like a cat slyly purring, "that's our little plan. Now—*strip!"*

Theo obeyed, as he'd always wanted to. Standing naked before them both, quivering a little nervously, being looked at lovingly by one and sardonically by the other, he felt all his years of towing a line—the masculine line, the "worker" line, the Party line—all those things which he knew now were just cages he'd learnt to build round himself, to gird himself with as if they were his skin—he knew now that he could break out of them all. He felt like an initiate into a secret and sacred society, like a shaman about to undertake a journey of discovery and the finding of power. Too, though, there was the happy feeling of *perversion*, of being *forced* into this perversion by two cruel, perverted girls, one of whom would gladly castrate him if he paid her enough, who played at it now as she shaved the hair off his face, his legs, his arms and chest, then applied the hot wax she'd brought to force him further from his ugly, hairy privileges and make him prettier than she was. Rouging his cheeks, lining his eyes, enveloping them in silvery shadow, gowning and corseting his body in the pretty, slutty outfit, fitting him with a jet black, bob-length wig to make him a cross between

Clara Bow and Theda Bara, Johanna chuckled more kindly than before. This boy she'd long teased didn't mind this prettiness, loved it with the thrill of the temptress he'd always wanted to be; when he pursed his lips to receive the blessings of the blue-black lipstick, it was almost a kiss.

Katya could barely contain herself, looking at him transformed, transfigured. He smiled, seductively, realizing the power she'd known in tempting him, feeling the blood flowing through him as through nymph-like butterfly's wings, still soft and wet from the chrysalis. She wanted him. And he wanted her. But, he wanted her in a different way than he'd ever wanted her before. It was cooler, easier, more melting than stiff. He longed not now to push inside her, to know her inner mystery which he, the boy, lacked and sought to know. Whether he'd been the "rapist" or the "raped" in their games of the last decade, he'd always felt his masculinity there, sticking out from him, the channel of all his desire—either as his weapon of dominance, or the strained, mocked token of his thwarted mastery. Not now, though. Now, it was blended into his body's totality, but one aspect of the energy he felt headily coursing through his veins. He wanted now to take her *into* him, and melt them both together. The instant he looked in the mirror above the washbasin, with Katya behind him, smiling, he understood that he was not this barren, acrid beak that had to push into someone else. He was a universe unto himself, and he could welcome her, Johanna, and the whole world of boys and girls in, knowing he could handle their roughness along with the smooth. He had something beautiful in his gut, he realized suddenly—and he wanted to share it.

For a moment, he wondered to that scene so long ago enacted in this very flat, between his love and his sister, that time Katya and Johanna had allowed him into their intimacy, to witness their perverse and natural union. He'd been a man, then—a boy, really—condemned by fear of himself to be an observer. Now, he felt he could join them, as a comrade in the flesh, in the warmth of gentle, thrilling decadence. Let the Communists make this Berlin a Gulag! Let the Nazis come and plunge it all into a new Dark Age! They all might die, and *soon*; but they would not have gone to their graves not knowing what it was to live . . .

"You look prettier than I thought you would," Johanna smiled, admiring Theo, and herself for making him who he now was, sitting there in his glory in the darkened suite. "I'll tell ya, little girl, I could almost kiss you . . ."

Then, with great purpose, and gleeful abandon, the three queer beauties left the flat, to go out into the last night of an era, dancing along the pavement to the red-curtained, greenishly-glowing grotto where they could forget quotidian ugliness and *dream*. Theo strode proudly in, with Katya and Johanna on each arm, to find the only men in the place who flashed it were the small jazz combo they swore was the same one who'd serenaded them years before from the flat below. A black pretty boy from the Camaroons, a gypsy bedecked as a Turkish Sufi, two French faggots in sequins and sparkles, and a stunning, bare-chested Nordic strongman, with a flower in his long hair—this was the combo, and their music was wild and sweet. But other than they, all in the place were women or those who strove to be, some pretty, some shy, some manly and fierce in the gloom. The walls were painted in green-tinted shellac, the tables rickety, but clothed in glorious vermilion tablecloths, and all was cigarettes and ashtrays, girlie drinks or bottles of strong beer. The women of body and the women of choice all danced together, many times couples of tough, short-haired *Bubis* and their pretty *Mädchen* loves, sometimes combinations of subtler variations of these. There were the Daddies, older butches who mannishly cuddled their younger beloveds. There were nefarious, shady Sharpers mingling here and there with ragged cigarettes hanging from their mouths and mean-looking jackknives hanging from their belts, in suit jackets or sharp skirts—or both in seamless combination. There were Garçonnes with their androgynous neck ties and bowl-cuts, who seemed almost as the young faggots Theo had danced with once in A Blue Moon in that lost era of half a decade past. Many of these hung on the arms of the Dodos, sophisticated and powerful women, young and middle-aged, whose immaculate, dark hair curled into Gypsy *Titus-kopfs*, their faces ivory with powder, their eyes bespectacled or monocled. Couples of these two styles, Dodos and Garçonnes, were almost always an item, an almost stereotype (Johanna laughed softly to Theo) that the two would be paired. But it was the elegant and dazzling Scorpions who dominated the scene—any of them a dead-ringer for Olga Rado from Weirauch's trilogy—tempting the young Gamines in their sexy, street urchin outfits—tempting, too, the ugly Tadpole wallflowers longing from the shadows. Even the bisexual call-girls, the Gougnettes who came and went, were tempted to fawn on these striking, Dianic goddesses, and serve them gladly for free.

And more than one of the straight Nuttes, those flapper-girls who came for the exotic, hep thrill of this dive—tourists, really, in such a place—even some of these straight girls gave the Scorpions the eye.

Johanna stood tallest and strongest and most beautiful of all the Scorpions, and Theo and Katya felt proud to be at her side. But all three felt a wealth in the human experience and variety round them in such an old, new style of Kaschemmen as this, one of the unlicensed, underground bars that stayed open well past Berlin's 3am closing-time. This one was as criminal as any other such establishment; but it was almost unique in that the criminals here were all Hot Sisters—the unregistered prostitutes and the drug dealers and the gangsters and the confidence women—a dozen types here, and easily a hundred people—plump or muscular or frail or diminutive, young or old or middle-aged, pretty or plain or ugly—or hotly, compellingly repulsive—all brazen and dark and full of life. The loners, looking to score, and the couples and triples and all—all defied the order of *burgerlich,* bourgeois society. Women who were once men, transvestites like Theo now, snuggling next to women so mannishly dressed as to pass almost as heterosexual lovers for the women that now hung on them. And here and there, as queer culture had flowered and diversified, there were even more subversive things—butch *Bubis* with effeminate ones, and couples of each kind; whole conjugal families of foursomes and fivesomes ranging from the very young to the very old; small groups and couples and individuals so androgynous they could have passed in the gay-boy circles as easily as here; and trios like Theo, Katya, and Johanna—all femmes in their way, held together by a subtle but gradually evident power-relation. So much here, defying the stereotypes that even many of the underground Berliner Hot Sister counter-cultures enshrined.

The light was low, a few garish chandeliers and the candles on the tables providing the whole of the illumination. But, to Theo, the shadows only made the women here more glorious, as Katya was glorious, in the darkness that softened the careworn cast of her visage, the worry lines and the emptiness that had so long taken her eyes, the frown that had long suggested itself even when she was laughing. And the wrinkles and syphilitic blemishes that marred Johanna, all were gone in the gloom. The night, Theo realized, was their friend. It was when all things were magical again, mysterious, and beautiful. It seemed no mistake that the symbol of the Nazis, the enemies of all this glorious and decadent darkness, was the swastika, the ancient symbol of the sun. The day was their world, where all things were laid bare, without beauty, without wonder, desiccated in the day's unforgiving glare. Safety, and sanity, these were the paranoid blessings of a world of light; it was in the world of the dreaming, of the night, that freedom lay.

People knew Johanna here, and Katya, too. Some came to fawn on them, some to bear-hug them as long lost sisters, and a few glared at them as if in challenge. These last, Johanna said, were old tops she knew from long ago, people she'd played with during her first years in this scene in the years before the war, when she did not wield the whip, but rather submitted to it. She smiled to them in bygone reverie, glancing from one to the other to the other, inviting them as an elder generation would have done with a folding fan aflutter, her face hid behind, in some parlour of a lost, mysterious, repressedly sexy Victorian age. They each seemed to know the signals and codes of that Victorian fan; but rather than come over to her, they each walked, one-by-one, into the darkened back room.

Johanna looked deliciously to her proteges, and pulled them slightly toward her.

"D'you know who those people were, darlings?" she said sultrily.

Katya squinted perplexed. Those dominas were before her time here. Theo was clueless as a newborn babe.

"I owe each of those women a debt," she smiled, "a debt of honour They were the people who made me who I am. They *trained* me, darlings. At first, like a dog; and then, like a hunter's falcon. Without them, there would be no Johanna; nor, I dare say, would there be pretty Katya—or pretty, pretty Theo."

They did not understand, but each of them looked to the darkened threshold of the back room. Katya began to anticipate what might happen back there, how her longtime mistress might choose to *pay* her debt of honour. Theo did not know what to think; but he was becoming painfully curious.

"Will you both do me the honour," Johanna pronounced, "of doing you an honour?"

"Do you mean—?"

"Yes, Katya, *meine lieblich sklavin*. I want to give you a night to remember me by. And, maybe, just maybe . . . someone to . . . see after you . . . when I'm gone."

Johanna looked away, sipping her Vana Tallinn and champagne, a mixed drink named for the symbol of her enemies, a little on the tepid side, so she drank it slowly. She looked through the dancing women on the sawdust-strewn floor to the black hole where her three once-lovers had disappeared, and waited a few moments, as if for some cue from the darkness. She must have received it, then, for she took both of her protégés in tow, and led them through the weaving bodies into the darkness, where they, too, disappeared.

The back room was surprisingly vast, its walls enshrouded by shadow, so it seemed even vaster. Suspended from the high ceilings were several trusses and rope-trellises and sets of chains and manacles, and on the walls were X-shaped St. Andrew's Crosses and a padded saw-horse or two, which Katya knew, and Theo guessed, were meant for a Prussian, boarding school discipline. A few women were bound amidst these contraptions, being tormented by steady lovers or lovers-for-the-night. But there were still two suspension apparatuses yet free. Johanna breathed that these had been "reserved" for Katya and Theo, by the deliciously sadistic Goddess of Chance. She brought the two to the three women, whose features (as everything here) were fuzzy and darkened. She smiled to each, and kissed each on the cheeks, *de la Francaise.* They kissed her back, then stood there, as imposing as ebony Amazon totems from some lost and ancient Dahomey kingdom, deep below the Sahara.

One of the women was dressed in the drag of a successful bourgeois, modest, tasteful suit, tie, proper shoes and spats, a watch fob and chain. Another was dressed as a workman, in the dirty, grey overalls Theodor himself would have worn a decade ago. The third was dressed, oddly, in the garb of an SA stormtrooper, complete with the goofy, frumpy bill-cap and black suspenders and shiny sable boots Katya and Theo had long learnt to hate. This last woman was the most androgynous of all, with a platinum-blonde bowl-cut and a natural moustache which she'd thickened with wax and shaped into a pencil. Katya thrilled at being topped by such a trinity, but feared them, too. Theo, who was just starting to get it all, trembled almost visibly—especially confused by the Brownshirt, wondering if the garb was meant as parody or the genuine article.

Even though he felt very wedded to his faggotry, and Katya's, as signs of a greater underground culture which, almost by nature, opposed the right wing; even so, Theo knew well that gays were everywhere in Germany. Even the Nazi thug of thugs, the SA leader Ernst Rohm, was said to take gay lovers. So, this third Garçonne of the sadist triumvirate was dubious and frightening. Not that any of the three didn't inspire a certain fear. Katya gave into it, instantly, as Johanna took her by her leash of silken scarves, knelt in homage before her mentors, and handed over her slave for their pleasure. Theo shivered in confusion, standing there with his leash of black pearls hanging down, held in his own, trembling hands. Johanna looked to him, and drew him close.

"This is an honour I do you, Theodor," she whispered, "but, too, an honour you do me. I don't want you to feel obligated, in any way. I know this is beyond what you've ever done. But, know I trust these women, and have trusted them, with my very life. They shan't hurt you . . . But, Theo, your consent is sacrosanct to me. I know Katya will do anything I wish; she *chooses* to do that, always. But you, Theo, you and I are not wedded as Katya and I. We have no compact, no contract, no agreement between us. . . . I grant you this honour, Theodor, because—because I love you."

"I love you, too," he breathed.

She pulled him toward her and kissed him on both cheeks, refraining from a deeper kiss out of concern for his health. He instantly took her cheeks in his hands, and kissed her deeply, his tongue massaging hers, and every part of her mouth and lips. He pulled away to look at her; she smiled to him tenderly.

"Thank you, Theodor," she breathed.

"Thank *you—meine Domina, meine Göttin—meine Johanna.*"

He put his leash in her hand of his own accord, and bowed when she handed it on.

Giving a gift both to her most ancient loves, and to her loves of the last decade she gave the former in tribute, Johanna stepped aside to let the triumvirate do their magic. The three consulted together, as if rugby players in a huddle, as if generals over a strategy, as if doctors in an operating theatre. Then, deciding, they went to work, the bourgeois, the worker, and the fascist producing a long sheet of latex rubber from somewhere, and the first two began wrapping Katya in it, mummifying her and then suspending her in the corner. Meanwhile, the fascist took Theo in her wiry arms and laid him on a hammock of silky rope, face down, his arms and legs spread-eagle, secured to the corners with leather cuffs. The faux Nazi (or was she real?) then tied a black silken scarf round Theo's eyes, gracefully, not disturbing the bob-wig or for a moment dispelling the simulacrum of Theo's womanhood. Soon Katya had been completely mummified in the latex, her nostrils filled with nought but the enticing scent of rubber she'd long had a fetish for, leaving her more immobilized than even the wet-pack in the sanatorium. Her eyes were blinded, her lips enshrouded, her fingers and toes wrapped tight in the sheath. Only a part round her nose was open, to allow her precious breath in and out, the flap moistening till sweat-like droplets formed there. Somebody's firm hand gently brushed these away from time to time.

Hands, everywhere, then nowhere. This was the two lovers' universe for what seemed eternity. Then, by their ears, hot-breathed, sultry voices intoned, German in several accents, lilting in the sexy way German could sound when the subject was *bumsen.*

To Katya, the voices said: "D'you *fear*, little girl? Being *left* here, like *this?* D'you *long* for the feel of our strong hands upon you—coming through the rubber? *Feel* it, little girl? We've left you so *helpless* you can't even *beg* . . ."

To Theo, the voices said: "D'you *long,* little girl? Is your little snatch *wet* with excitement, and wonder? What shall we *do* to you? How shall we have *our way with you* . . . ?"

Katharina revisited all her horrid helplessness, suspended—just like *this*—above the hydrotherapy chamber on that sterile ward in the darkest places in her memory. She'd blocked out years from her life, swinging there, and all at once in a desire charged with terror, these dark places emerged from oblivion and flooded her mind. She recalled every moment, every second of the years she'd spent on that horrible ward, and would have screamed out loud if not gagged by the rubber sheath. The humming of her thwarted screams massaged her face and travelled throughout her body, till the sound and the sensation were one. In that tingly terror, there was more sensation: firm hands everywhere, pairs beyond counting. A whisper in her ear, the voice she was sure was the Nazi, telling her the whole bar had been invited to be her tormentors, to taste and touch and fuck their fill of her. A space opened up, and a waft of air made her realize her pussy had been opened up like a flower to be ravaged by a swarm of bees. Tongues flittered, fingers danced, fists soon pushed their way in, violating her blind and helpless body—and all the while her screams hummed amidst orgasmic groans, writhing within her mummy-wrappings like a fish on an angler's hook.

Theodor heard the voices calling, heard the worker-bitch

calling him a sell-out revolutionary, heard the bourgeois-bitch mocking his origins, his lack of taste and culture, heard the nazi-bitch cackling derision at him for his forsaken manhood. The voices of his tormentors of flesh merged with the nameless, nebulous tormentors of his darkest mind, the voices he'd heard since he'd lost all faith and hope in the bowels of a French prison. The voices merged, the women who fucked him now, and the devils who tormented him always, till he quivered and shook with the tortures of them both. But the many hands caressed him as thoroughly as they did Katya, hands pulling and playing with the strap of his silky underwear, but not removing it. His cock, hard and pulsing, was pressed up against his flesh—rendered now an enlarged clit, more than a few whispered to him. He would learn to come with it harder than he'd ever come over his years of "misusing" it. Rough hands, and soft, each had their fun massaging and slapping and pinching his long clit, pushed up tight against his body so that he felt it all through his hips and gut, and the feeling he felt earlier that evening expanded like an impregnated womb within him. All of it, all the hands and tongues and grazing fingernails began to build in him something beyond the anticipation he'd known over his twenty-seven years in a male body. He drew it all in, feeling it raging inside him like a demon, or a legion of demons—dancing and bursting and trying to flee his body as if commanded by scores of dark, saintly exorcists—they who had possessed him in the first place. For the first time in his life, he felt his soul, palpably inside him . . .

Their tormentors brought them together, then, pulling the suspension-pulleys across tracks in the ceiling, smashing them together in the middle of the room. All eyes were on the two, now, the most adored souls in the room—even the other tops and bottoms pausing from their activities to grant the slaves their fealty. Still blind, still uncertain of any of their surroundings, they did not know into whose bodies they were being pushed. Johanna did the final honour of all the honours bestowed that night, and unmasked them so they looked to each other, eye to eye, nose to nose, as Maori warriors were said to do; their eyes widened and blurred in mute communion.

"Now, my darlings," Johanna said, as if the last words at a deathbed side, "I shall send you to the *stars* . . . *Remember, darlings; remember **me** . . .*"

She stuck a device originally designed in the nineteenth

century, a medical treatment for the ill effects of ruined orgasms Victorian wives suffered at the unskilled hands of their errant husbands, which had been but recently reclaimed in a way to emancipate the fairer sex from needing husbands at all. She stuck this wand between Theo and Katya, and released the wound-up spring within it, so that it vibrated in a powerful buzz. The two clitorises were like two ends of an electric wire, positive and negative charges on both ends, winding in a sustained current loop, sparking like Tesla coils in the labs of all those mad scientists haunting modern cinema—all on the delicious verge of creating *Life.*

"Hold it *in,*" Johanna hissed like a comet—*"Hold it **in**—till the last **possible** moment . . ."*

All the energy of the room seemed to channel through that rod into them both, their muffled screams only intensifying it all. There was no longer male or female, straight or queer, flesh or machine, this or that. There was now only energy—***Eros***—the one power that no government could ever steal away. It built up and up and up as the cheers and the laughter roared round them; it swelled and swelled to explosion in the crash of breaking glass.

Though Katya and Theo were lost now, swirling in worlds of their own, spinning in a whirlwind of sensation and energy and light, the rest of the club left the back room to see what had made the noise which punctuated the muffled ecstasies of their collective bottoms. Johanna alone stayed near them, making sure they were all right, coaxing them back from the Beyond with kisses and caresses and softest words. But her three butch-top mentors, and most all the rest, gathered round the brick that had broken through Pandora's Box's only window and toppled a table, the candle atop it catching fire to the oily, liquor-stained tablecloth and feeding on all the alcohol puddling on the floor over the last hours. There were shouts outside, men's shouting, drunken jeers declaring—**"HAPPY NEW YEAR YOU QUEER DEFECTIVE BITCHES!!"**

Some women ran out of the bar, and started a street fight with the Brownshirts outside. The sirens of the Bullen and the fire brigades followed. By the time they arrived, the Brownshirts had scattered, leaving the dykes in the bar to be hauled away almost to a woman. Though Weimar law did not penalize lesbianism as it did male homosexuality, at least not in letter, a host of charges were trumped up that night by bored and ugly Bullen, including for the proprietresses of the place for code violations, a lack of proper licenses, even attempted arson. The bar just now called Pandora's Box was going to have to close again, as many times before, not opening ever again under that name.

Johanna cut her two lovers down, and spirited their bewildered, exulted bodies away, out a back cellar door she knew from long nights past, just in the nick of time.

Chapter 19

The joy of New Year's Eve of 1930 did not last very far into the wee hours of New Year's Day, 1931. Johanna was hung over, the dawn's light stirring her early, and she was tortured by nausea and a vicious headache most of the day. In a sense, she never got over that hangover. For the triumphant perversity of last night's (and last year's) celebration was never to be revisited. Johanna did not play with Katya and Theo with any of those dommes again. And as if some glorious last hurrah of health and sanity, that last night of the decade marked the last moment Johanna was free of the ugliness of full-blown syphilis. She gave up her apartment in Spandau, and curled up in a ball of pain on Katya's floor. There she lay for the next three months, drinking constantly, smoking hashish and opium, sniffing and shooting cocaine and heroin, and downing a host of multicoloured pills—all in the vain hope of forestalling the agonies which raged at her like furies from the netherworld. Theo for the first time felt the full brunt of her angers and hates, dodging her curses and even her blows. For Katya, it was a more familiar strain—not that this made it any easier.

After a while, as spring came in lemon yellow sharpness and derangement, the increasingly disfigured and debilitated Johanna began to beg her closest friends to help her end it all.

"I DON'T WANT IT!" she screamed—**"I DON'T WANT THIS!!"**

And she cursed and cried, tearing up the room, smashing plates and vases, dealing her wrath on the books she'd collected over a lifetime of feminist defiance. She even set fire to them one night, her English novels and her German novels and her French—throwing *Herland* and all the novels of Grete von Urbanitzki and Willa Cather and Kate Chopin, her Virginia Woolf and her Djuna Barnes and her Anna Elisabet Weirauch, her Amazon and her Colette and her Louise M. Gagneur, all her poetry and pornography, her Sappho and her Sade and her Dolorosa—in a smouldering pile on the carpeted floor. Katya and Theo barely managed to snuff out the flames before the fire brigade would have had to be called.

"She's in Hell," Katya told Theo, both of them sitting like children on the blackened, torched and patchy Persian rug as their elder sister slept the sleep of the dead on the twin mattress they now all shared together. She'd drunk a whole fifth of vodka in but a few hours; only such excesses could dull the pain. "The one thing she's always feared—as long as *I've* known her, at least—is to lose control. She can't face being powerless. . . . Shit, schätzelein! She's spent her entire career trying to escape that wretched feeling. And, now . . . ?"

Theo looked at her solemnly.

"We should help her, liebschin," he said.

There was a long pause.

"Theo—what are you saying?"

"You know precisely what I'm saying."

Katya looked away. She herself had spent a lifetime trying to escape the urge her friend now felt overtaking her. It was against everything that kept Katya alive to concede to the Demon Death Its prize.

"It might be our fate, too, darling," he said quietly.

She looked back to him, then away again. Her eyes found her old friend, sleeping corpse-like there in the grey afternoon.

"Yes. Yes, Theo. I know that."

"She's asked us. . . . What else would a true comrade do? What else can *we* do?"

Katya nodded.

"How," she asked, "should we do it?"

"Well . . . that's up to her, I suppose."

They sat a moment. Then, they wept.

Johanna had laughed often that her career as a tormentor of men had revolutionary potential. She laughed lately of infecting as many Brownshirts with syphilis as she could before she went. (She might have done this already, to one, or two, or ten of those ugly bastards—who could know?) She half-thought to get a stick or two of dynamite, and hijack a taxi, driving it straight into the Reichstag during a parliament session, and take out as many ministers as she could in a blaze of glory and gasoline. Now, though, she wondered.

A rope? A knife? A pistol? Morphine? Cyanide?

All these things were entertained, openly, with the loving support of her friends—however hard it was to hear and say. In the end, though, it was the death of her favourite poet which beckoned. The ancient poetess—the first, and best. Sappho, mourning a young Phaon's spurning, throwing herself off the Leucadian cliffs into the Aegean.

"Let's take a walk, darlings," she smiled to them of a

midnight in earliest April. She'd taken no drink, no pills that afternoon. She'd spent the evening making love to Katya—down on her knees, worshipping her perennial submissive, giving her a taste of what she'd herself long known. Katya looked down at her as she showered her feet with kisses, and wept to think of how she wished to be down on *her* knees, touching her lips to her longtime love's syphilitic blemished ankles and calves, to dare fate and bury herself in her mistress' sex, if for but one last time. But Johanna knelt, and Johanna worshipped, as Jesus had done to his Apostles to show the path of true leadership. She'd wanted to give her someone to take care of her, had hoped that proud trinity at Pandora's Box would be a trio of mistresses for her most beloved slave. But those women were not friends to Katya, and would never be. One had left Berlin; another had been raped and murdered by SA, they said; the last had fallen further than anyone could conceive, and had married a man— a stuffy Lutheran minister connected to the Christian Trade Unions in Munich. All this in four short months. Weimar was dying. You could hear its death rattles echoing from the rafters of the tenements and the tunnels of the subway. Johanna would die before it, her own breathing raspier and raspier by the night. And before she went, she would give this last token of love to Katya, granting her her own wings before she flew away.

"Now," she said, as Katya kissed her, defiant of the danger, full on the lips after their ritual, "now, my darling, the master has bowed to the slave. The slave, who is now a master. I . . . set you free, my love . . ."

And then, as the clock struck the witching hour on that blustery spring night that had not yet shed its winter, Johanna dressed to the nines, as did Katya and Theo—all dandies, all fabulous and artful, in masculine, *Mannweib* drag they'd toyed with during Fasching celebrations of years past—and the three friends walked, parasols and walking-sticks in hand, to that bridge over the Spree they'd walked a thousand times before—the place where, ten years ago, Katharina had first seen the young clown Erik hanging suspended from a rope and sexily escaping a straitjacket—the place where, just three years and three months later, Theodor, his mother and sister, had together scattered his father's ashes, watching in the sunset as all the old man had been dissolved into the current. They stood there now, the three of them, Theo on one side, Johanna on the other, Katya, as always, in the middle.

The suit Johanna wore was black velvet and tight, her

blazer's pockets, her vest's and slacks', loaded down with bricks and scrap coal stolen from the rathskeller of the old Black Tie. This was as she wanted it.

"Well, then, darlings," she said, "time waits for no man."

And before anyone could say anything, before any embarrassing speeches or droll black humour could be enunciated, Johanna pecked each of them on the cheek, gave each a resounding slap on the ass. Then—

"Johanna!"

Theo held Katya back from following her longtime lover over the railing.

Chapter 20

The summer was high, but the temperatures seemed frozen, like an ice field in an ironic Hades. Katya and Theo mourned their departed as only a widow and widower could. That space in the bed, that indentation in the pillow, those stains on the sheets. Johanna's rocker, so close a cousin to the one that had rocked there in eras past, her throne forever, seemed to creak at night now, ghostly. Her old Victrola, whose platters were scratched and warped, whose needle was long worn down. Those bottles of vodka, bottles of gin, bottles of Russian champagne and Estonian Vana Tallinn piled in a solemn collection in the corner, like trophy harts from a lifetime's hunting. Her mirror of pressed butterflies, discoloured by years of white powder, still clinging to the scratches and the cracks. Tight lace garters and yellow strips of rubber Katya could neither feel again on her skin nor taste again in her teeth, for the knowledge of the purpose they'd served, scattered in forgotten corners of the rooms. All was quiet, afternoonlike, no matter what the hour. All was a tomb in their once gay slum salon.

Summer passed, as the spring had, with a whimper, not a bang. Communists were outdoing the Nazis in the electoral campaigns; but to two anarchists, who were moving anew toward surrealism as a protest, and a reflection, of the world round them, such was no good news. The mark again plummeted, and the breadlines grew longer and longer. Katya didn't move from her bed for three long weeks in July. Theo, who felt again that he was followed, by spirits as much as men, hearing both shouting at him from the sewers and the sky, managed miraculously over those days and nights to leave the flat at least once a day, carting his suitcase full of marks that Katya had long withdrawn from the bank, to buy a few loaves of bread and a jug of wine. His mind entwined round every stimulus, every hint and echo of the world outside the flat, from the crying children in the apartments just at the threshold of the street to the high-pitched cackles, hard to identify, yet Theo had always known them, in a flat somewhere between the street level and his own. His spirits declined every moment, every morning walk, every sleepless night. The despair, the utter absurdity grew intolerable the first broiling day of August, when a group of kids no older than elementary-schoolers took to fighting by the score in the street outside his tenement, tangling in hopeless imitation of their elders, without even the insane sense of politics.

A rock flew by Theo's head, and he ducked as if it were a bullet.

"Jesu Maria!" he spat in hopeless contempt. "What the hell you kids doin' anyway?! Can't you let an old man walk in peace?!"

"You ain't so old."

Theo spun round to see a fellow—or was it a girl?—leaning in a neighbouring door frame, with a bottle of beer in *ihre Hand.*

"Here," sie said. "Ya wanna drink this, man?"

"What? I,er—why don't *you* drink it?"

"Bumsen! I ain't drinkin' this piss! Alcohol's stupid!!"

Theo looked at the androgynous kid before him quizzically. He knew he was only a little older than sie was, a decade and a few years on the outside (he used the gender-neutral term in his head without thinking). But generations seemed to separate them somehow. Sie was shorter than he, maybe half a foot shorter. Sie dressed in ragged clothes, patchy, a threadbare overcoat of navy blue and black denim trousers, stained with dirt and bicycle grease. Ihr face, *ihr Gesicht,* was black-framed spectacles, a sneer of joyful contempt, *ihre Haare* short but wildly uncombed, sticking out blondish and brown and red from beneath a newsboy cap. *Ihre Füße* were clad in steel-toed leather, a little bulky for *ihre Füße,* a little clownish in aspect—though he could see sie could give a hell of a kick with them, if there was a mind to. Military boots, left over from the War, by the look of them. Rescued from the trash? Or, stolen?

"Well," Theo said, "why don't ya just spill the beer out, then?"

"Oh," sie smiled prettily and tough, "that'd be wasteful, eh Papa? Here, pal—drink it for me, huh? It's only just been opened. Actually a good brand, so they say . . ."

Theo half suspected the kid had dumped ihre own piss in it, or maybe slipped in some kind of a mickey. But he was too dejected and confused to care.

"Sure," he said, and took it from the kid, downing the whole bottle in one long swallow.

"Thanks, Vati," sie giggled—*"LOOK OUT!!"*

Theo ducked in time, as a brick flew over his head into the glass of the window beside sie.

"Bumsen! Arschloch!! Take *THAT!!!"*

And sie flung the empty bottle straight at the golden head

of a senior, uniformed member of the *Hitler Jugend*. The curse was returned, along with the crash of broken glass.

Theo spun round, still crouching down. Suddenly, the street fight made sense. A little more than half the kids in the street were Hitler Youth boys. The other half were teenagers of all genders, who wore no uniforms. Yet, in a way, they *were*. All of the others, now that Theo saw it clearly, were dressed in mismatched, patchy, hand-me-down outfits, many wearing boots a lot like the person next to him now.

"What the hell's goin' on out here??"

Sie was not wasting time; sie had repositioned in Theo's door frame, and seeing Theo's paralysing confusion, was pulling him in over the threshold. Sie slammed the door shut, then crouched down to look through the mail slot in the door to the scene outside. A flurry of rocks, bottles, and eggs pummelled the door with almost machine-gun staccato.

"Reinhardt!" sie cried through the slot—"Quietschend! C'mon, guys—over here!!"

Two fellows broke away from the rest as the Hitler Youth retreated and the Bullen sirens sounded. A group of the motley kids chased the *Hitler Jugend* across the scrapyard outside the long disused factory. The two older fellows pushed their way into Theo's tenement's door, and stood with them there.

"Ha ha!" sie laughed, clapping *ihre Hände* on the young fellows' backs. "You guys fucked up that sandwich-board kid—but *good! Wunderbar!!*"

"Yeah," laughed the fellow called Reinhardt, a trim, slight fellow with umber hair, cut uneven, with little pais-like curls round his ears, "thanks, Kanalratte. You did good coverin' us."

The other fellow smiled, but said nothing.

"Just *look* at that fuck!" Kanalratte sneered triumphantly, peering again through the slot—"He don't even *know!*"

"What don't he know?" Theo asked.

"C'mon down here, Vati."

Theodor crouched down, gazing at what Kanalratte pointed out. Standing around with a puffy, blackened eye, some Aryan type of an age and stature between Hitler Youth and Brownshirt was marching round in circles at the far corner. His sandwich-board sign declared: "ACHTUNG! ARBEITER HUTEN LUGEN JUDEN!" which Theo took to mean a rather illiterate notice for workers to beware of "Jewish Lies." But then, he looked again, and saw the word "JUDEN" was modified in black paint over the crude stencil. It now said "JUGEND," and affixed above it was one of the symbols of the Hitler Youth. **The idiot!** Theo laughed, and his new companions joined him. The back of his sandwich-board declared proudly now—***Workers Beware of [Hitler] Youth Lies!***—and the fool didn't even know it!

"That's why sie's the 'sewer rat,'" Reinhardt laughed, rubbing his knuckles, bruised on the Nazi's bruised eye. "Sie crawls right beneath where you think sie is—and fucks up all yer shit before you even know sie was there!"

"Very good!" Theo laughed. "That's cold as hell!"

"The ox won't even know he's been canvassing for our side," the quiet fellow with the "squeaky" name chuckled wryly, "till he goes back to HQ and takes that stupid billboard off."

"And," Reinhardt added, "he'll probably get paid for his time with a kick in his backside, once his mates read what he's been advertising."

"So," Theo said, suddenly gay again for the first time in seasons, "you folks say, 'our side'?"

"Yeah, Opa!" Kanalratte giggled. "See our patches?"

Theo looked to their overcoats. In a different place on each of them, the lapel, or the breast, or the sleeve, was sewn a rendering of a little white flower.

"An Edelweiss?" Theo asked.

"That's right, *alter,*" Kanalratte said; "we're the Edelweiss Pirates!"

"What's that?"

They explained. There were just a few of them now, maybe twenty, maybe fifty round Berlin. Most had been members of the Hitler Youth, or the Girls' version of it, the *Bund Deutscher Mädel.* All had become disillusioned with those groups, and the politics of racism and urges to sickly chastity and purity those groups imposed. Now, these radical kids were beating up their former comrades in the streets, disrupting *Hitler Jugend* meetings, and painting anti-Nazi slogans on every wall and billboard hoarding they could.

Theo invited the three up to the flat, just till the heat died off down there, and sat down with them with all the enthusiasm he would have sat down to a Communist Youth Brigade meeting ten years ago. This was exciting! He lit a smoke for himself and poured himself a drink, offering them both cigarettes and gin—but found they neither smoked nor drank. He offered to brew some coffee instead, and found this much more amenable.

"So," he smiled, "you cats were all in the Nazi youth groups before?"

"When I was *five!*" laughed Reinhardt.

"Yeah," mused Kanalratte, "sometimes you're foolish when you're young."

"How old are you?"

"Fourteen," Reinhardt said.

"Thirteen," said Kanalratte.

"I'm all of seventeen," smiled the Cheshire Cat Quietschend. "But I was never in it. I'm 'racially impure,' you know."

"What's that mean?"

"His Vati's Japanese," Kanalratte explained.

"Yeah," laughed Quietschend. "Although, I hear talk from the scumbag Nazi thinktanks that my dad's side might get 'grandfathered in' to the Aryan race. The sauschwobs need 'em for allies, you know. Funny how much your ancestors' blood can 'evolve' to 'higher' forms, if warms bodies need to spill it in the present generation. You know how it is in our brave, new world, chum—only the 'purest' sheep'll get to be slaughtered in the trenches of the next war."

They all laughed.

"How many of you guys are there round Germany?"

They looked at each other.

"Who knows?" Kanalratte said. "Hopefully, the thing'll grow and grow. I mean, a lotta kids join up with the Nazi outfits because of bicycles."

"And camping," Reinhardt smiled. "A chance to leave the city, and get lucky with some pretty frauleins in the bushes when the 'scoutmasters' ain't lookin'."

"Not just frauleins, though," laughed Kanalratte. "Whatever's clever, y'know."

"The more, the merrier," Reinhardt agreed.

They chatted on, over the next hour, and Katya arose to the once-familiar sound of young, tough, giggly talking. When she saw the three Pirates sitting around, their eyes wired on the second kettle of coffee Theo brewed, she got a flashback to the kids she used to know, back round the Revolution in '18, when her great aunt took her to a demonstration in defiance of their family, introducing her to an on-and-off girlfriend of her butler, who spirited Katharina away for three days and nights, introducing her to anarchy and Sapphism in one glorious afternoon.

Katya told them the story, a story that in almost ten years, Theo had never heard. She told them of that, and many other stories of being younger, her own less than legal activities and her firm commitment to their being less than legal. She told them how she'd been thrown out of an elite private school right after her best therapist killed himself; how she'd been locked away for a season in a high-class bedlam and sterilized against her will; how her great aunt had helped break her out and how they'd run away to Switzerland during the War and lived amidst the crazy artists of the first wave of Dada; how she and her great aunt had imposed an exile on themselves and travelled to Paris and London and Tangiers and Mexico City and finally Chicago and New York before sneaking back into Germany via a Norwegian fishing boat on the Baltic—arriving back just in time for the German Revolution in 1918 and the fall of the hated Kaiser. She told swashbuckling tales of falsified identities and stowing away on ships, narrow escapes from the authorities of various countries, passing for French in Allied countries and Austrian in those of the Central Powers. She told them of wanting to start a commune someday, somewhere in this wide, crazy world, half-wanting to invite these new friends along.

The kids seemed impressed. They talked long and well as the afternoon drifted into evening, Kanalratte dropping away to parley with a stray, threadbare alley cat who had come through a hole in the wall, leaving the two young fellows to chat with the "old geezers" in a friendly, joyfully sarcastic way. Theo was painfully aware of the difference between himself and Katya, and these others, in style, in politics, in age—aware, painfully, by how little the differences actually were. The squeaky fellow began talking in a clever, silly way about "manoeuvres" his "acquaintances" "may or may not" be planning in the hill country of Switzerland. Manoeuvres, movements of little armies, armies in training, Quietschend laughed by degrees.

"Armies?" Katya inquired.

"Oh," Quietschend smiled quizzically, "so I've *heard.* Couldn't say for sure. Such things are *illegal*, you know."

"We wouldn't do anything *illegal*," Reinhardt smiled knowingly. "That would be—against the law."

"Gotta respect the law," Kanalratte chuckled to the cat,

petting its nearly bald crown as it nuzzled sie. "Without respect for the law, what d'you have?"

"Lawlessness," Reinhardt said, just shy of seriously. "Rowdiness. Hooliganism . . ."

"Nothin' like that in Switzerland," Quietschend smiled. "Ascona's a *civilised* place."

"Ascona?" Theo asked.

"Yeah, chum," Quietschend grinned, "you know the place?"

"Yeah, actually. I've got some friends who live there, last I checked. My friends Nadia and Sebastien. They've got a chalet there, I'm told. A collective house."

"Oh, there's a lot of those there, chum. Ever since Mounte Verita, y'know, the 'Hill of Truth,' was founded there—long before *we* were born. Betcha *you're* old enough to know about it, though."

For the second time, Theodor laughed at this reversal of the ageism he'd grumpily laid on these kids back in the street. "How would you know, sonny?" he snickered. "How old d'ya take me for anyway?"

"Oh, sixty—seventy easily."

"Surprise you ain't walkin' with a cane yet, pops," Reinhardt chuckled. "You must exercise real good."

Theo laughed, and gave up on it.

"So," he said instead, "Ascona's big for communes, then?"

"Oh, yeah, Vati," Quietschend said. "The land 'round there's like, mountains and the foothills of mountains. Alps are just north, y'know. My mum's land is useless for farming, almost useless for building—maybe a way-station for climbers, a lookout for rangers, maybe, but that's all you'd wanna build. But it's *ideal* for what *I* wanna do."

"What d'you wanna do?"

Quietschend smiled cryptically.

"Maybe, once I got to know ya, old man," he chuckled, "I'll let ya in."

Theo smiled and nodded.

"Aw, let 'im in!" Reinhardt enjoined—"let 'em both in!"

"Maybe," said Quietschend. Then, he leaned in to Katharina. "So, you've been interested in communes, eh, auntie?"

"Sure," Katharina said.

"Well, you know—there's some *nice* property up in the hills there, by Ascona. 'Least, I've *heard* as much. And Switzerland, you know. Stays outta wars, nice people, lovely sights. This property, auntie. No way to beat it."

Katya rolled with it.

"You lookin' to sell me a—a bill o' goods, there, Quietschend?"

"Who? *Me?* I wouldn't *dream* o' somethin' like that, auntie. I'm just sayin'. Switzerland—it's a good place to be."

Kanalratte was studying Theodor and Katharina, as well as *ihre Freunde*, from the corner with the stray cat. Sie seemed to be discussing them all with the cat, as a cat, in Cat. They purred to each other a while; then the stray cat disappeared again through the hole in the wall. Kanalratte got up.

"C'mon," sie said. "It's time to go."

Quietschend was still coyly half-selling his mother's land to Katya; Reinhardt got up with Kanalratte, but seemed unsure of whether to leave.

"Quietschend," Kanalratte said, "c'mon, man. It's time to go."

"Well—okay."

"Where you guys headin'?" Theo heard himself ask.

"Kinda far," Quietschend smiled. "You guys know the Underground?"

"You mean, the subway?" Katya said.

"That's right. You ever been?"

"We've lived in Berlin all our lives," Theodor said. "Of course we've been."

"No, man," Kanalratte corrected. "Have you ever *really* been?"

The two young, old people looked to each other quizzically; they drew a common blank.

"C'mon, pal," Reinhardt said, taking Theo by the arm, "get your coat and hat. And, some shoes you don't mind gettin' dirty."

"You too, auntie," Quietschend smiled, waving his arm as he got up. "You can use that ermine stole—you don't wanna wear that old thing out dancin' any more, eh?"

Theo and Katya smiled. This was the most adventurous they'd been in months, years, they both thought, and exchanged looks that confirmed each of them were thinking the same thought.

"What the hell?" they laughed in unison, and donned their "old folk" clothes. They followed the kids down an intricate series of alleys to a subway stop near the mid-town sections of Berlin. They followed the three over the turnstiles, past the hectors demanding their fares, past the commuters looking sombre and tired after their long day, then—and neither "old person" could really believe it as they did it—*right onto the tracks!*

"Gotta hurry there, *Große Opa, Große Oma!*" Kanalratte called over *ihre Schulter*—"else the train'll come, 'n' squish ya like rotten, billion-paper-mark eggs!"

They ran till they huffed and stumbled over the ties of the tracks, the hectors giving up on them, the tracks rumbling with the coming of a train.

Was this the end?

What an ending it would be!

As the tunnel darkened, their three new friends suddenly disappeared. Theodor and Katharina kept running, then halted in a confused huff, looking round them desperately.

"Where'd they go?!" Katharina demanded of the empty air.

"Here, old lady! C'mon in!!"

An arm seemed to come straight out of the wall; in the darkness, Katya grabbed the offered hand. She was pulled through a crack in the wall, seeming too narrow, but just wide enough. She put her arm out and grabbed Theo. Within instants, the train thundered by; but they were already inside . . .

Where they were was a large, stonewalled chamber, a storage chamber, disused and forgotten, dating back to when these tracks were first laid, decades ago. It hadn't been much thought of since the tunnels were dug. The pipes lining the ceilings leaked some strange, greenish substance in drips down to the stained, cement floor, cable-housings frayed and made a shambles by generations of rats gnawing at them. An old miner's lamp sat in a corner, providing the only light in the place, so all was long, dancing shadows, the far corners bathed in cobwebby darkness. But the room was not spare. It was well-furnished, actually, with a low table formed by an electrical spool, crates making a circle round it, several well-stocked bookshelves, even a dilapidated sofa mouldering along a wall. How had they stocked this place? And how had they kept it hidden from the rail road bulls and hectors who presumably were charged with keeping this place locked up?

Kanalratte was cagey about answering these questions. Reinhardt and Quietschend sat down at the table and picked up a game of chess where they'd apparently left off earlier in the day. Several other youths were in residence here, a pretty, dark-haired girl of maybe sixteen years with a large Star of David hanging defiantly from her neck, and two young boys, seeming no older than nine or ten, sharing a big bottle of bock beer in a corner, one platinum blonde, the other dark as night, his father a Senegalese soldier stationed in the Rhine valley during the Great War (he chuckled, in a Munich accent). Kanalratte cranked up an old, stolen Victrola, its horn dented and tarnished, to send a scratchy Louis Armstrong solo to dance through the chamber *in res media*. One bookshelf's lowest shelf was two dozen long-play albums, all American Jazz and Blues, all (they all said proudly) artists as black as Deutschland was white.

Katharina and Theodor stood a long moment in the midst of it all, as the kids settled down as if they did not plan to move for the rest of the night. Quietschend eyed them avuncular and amused after a moment, saying, "This is it, folks. Ain't nothin' else to see . . ."

Katya and Theo stood an awkward moment more; then, laughing, they collapsed onto the old, mouldy couch. Kanalratte cooked up some tea in a busted up kettle over a flame in a circle of a severed metal drum, right on the floor, the smoke leaving the room through mysterious gratings in the high ceilings. Once that had boiled, sie poured out some of it into a big, earthenware bowl, and shared it round. Theo found it the most potent tea he'd ever drunk, almost stinging his tongue. Katya felt a jolt from just a few sips, and watched with wonder as sie guzzled half the bowl, *ihre* bespectacled *Augen* almost popping from *ihr Gesicht* as sie sat back to enjoy the high fashioned from it.

After a time, the light began to flicker on the miner's headlamp. To the old folks' surprise, the two youngest boys scaled a small ladder in a dark corner, built into the wall beneath a rusty manhole, and stuck the thing on part of the exposed cables till they'd juiced it up again.

"You guys got quite the place here," Katya laughed.

"It's a cosy little mouse hole," Kanalratte yawned. "Sure beats the parents' house, or the boarding school."

"So, you're all 'emancipated,' as they say?" Theo said.

"That's right, daddy. We've all been on our own down here for months. And before here, it was somewhere else."

"You've got no other homes, then?"

"Who needs 'em? We take care of each other, and we've got a whole network o' places we can be."

"Squeaky here's got a 'proper' place," Reinhardt teased. "In the dormitories of the Polytechnic. He's our bourgeois relative."

"Bumsen," Quietschend chuckled. "There, you sauschwob bastard. Check*mate!*"

Reinhardt slammed his hand on the makeshift table and toppled all the pieces. Everyone laughed.

Theo and Katya wondered for a while, in this little forgotten space in the middle of the city they'd lived in all their lives, at these kids they never knew about. They half expected to be introduced to a new party, a new politic, perhaps a new religion. But once they got to the safety of the little mouse hole, they weren't explained to about anything. Having brought their new, old friends to their parlour, the Pirates seemed not even to notice them. Everyone could be here, if they were invited in—you were expected to take the hospitality at face value. Questions seemed almost rude.

Having lived the better part of ten years hep to the underground cultures of Weimar, radical political circles, queer, hidden dalliances, avant-garde artistry, and all the rest, Theodor and Katharina thought they'd seen it all. But these folks had escaped their notice, as they'd evidently escaped all things established and adult. History was not apparent to them, and they weren't apparent to history. Yet, here they were, a small but growing movement of anti-fascism (and anti-communism, too), in the hidden places of this same Berlin. They were young; they had no structured politics, no great knowledge of history. But they weren't crippled by the lack of these things. They were proud of it, stronger because of it. Nazism, socialism, communism, the whole mad mess of the last decade—none of this touched them. They needed no great theory or analysis to justify their rebellion against all the ugliness of Deutschland. They were rebellion incarnate—proof, Katya affirmed, and Theo mused wondrously, of the natural tendency in the human animal to rise up against evil, to affirm dignity, autonomy, and freedom.

They came back to the little hole in the wall, deep below Berlin, many times over the next weeks, meeting many of the Edelweiss Pirates round the city and having long conversations about the state of the world. Not all of them were runaways, but most of them were. They were from all classes, many ethnicities. But most were from the working classes, and all revolted against the culture of misery their elders were trying to impose on them, rejecting the lot tradition *and* most radicalism would have fated them with. They might have come from working stock, but they weren't about to cow-tow to the regimen of toil and discipline work and school and the churches—as well as the socialist, communist, and even a lot of the anarchist organizations—seemed committed to forcing on them. They were young and free. And, Katya and Theo thought, they were all quite beautiful . . .

Quietschend talked long and often about his mother's land in Switzerland, and the pals he and others had met there, mostly the same age and politics as they, and those mysterious "manoeuvres" his "acquaintances" "might or might not" be conducting there in the countryside. Theo and Katya wrote Sebastien and Nadia, their old comrades who still lived outside Ascona in Switzerland, reading between the lines of the code Katya had worked out with them years ago to find that yes, indeed, there were "some developments" in the countryside near their mountain chalet.

Maybe it was time to take a holiday . . .

Chapter 21

The holiday was a lift to Katya's and Theo's spirits, the second half of 1931 spent in Ascona, Switzerland, beginning with a pleasant, scenic train ride from the German heartland to the very foothills of the Alps, with three young comrades along for the ride. Passports and visas were got, though in this time between the wars (all of them knew, distantly, that another was coming—it was only a matter of time), the borders of contiguous European countries were not the hard stone walls of later years. Nobody questioned Reinhardt, Quietschend, and Kanalratte at the side of the two adults, who posed as their guardians in public, though they all laughed long and well on such silly subterfuges when in the privacy of their first class compartment. Their rendezvous was some place Quietschend knew, a stone's throw from his mother's land at the foot of the Alpine country, some place the quizzical young fellow said was a "cultural anomaly" run by a slightly drunken artist of Irish culture, though no Celtic blood flowed in her veins. A retreat the place was to be, their gateway to a further retreat, the chalet of their friends Sebastien and Nadia, who had lived for years now in connubial bliss, despite their internationally-recognized marriage license. Katya and Theo joked about how "married life" surely ruined most people, how they prided themselves on how they would never, ever marry. But Sebastien and Nadia had married for convenience, Sebastien's Swiss citizenship conferred on his Polish bride by the transaction, preventing deportation—and therefore no bad thing. They'd made up a new name for their household, which in the tradition of the Syndicalist Women's Union of years before, promised no blood-related children by the firm choice of the participants. They had taken up the position outlined in their friend Rudolf Rocker's writings—that human beings were called to be "race traitors"—active enemies of all domination, ethnic, class— and even *species.* These comrades of Katya's and Theo's had joined with a new surname, taken from the Russian word for "comrade"— the most fitting surname they could come up with. For comrades they were, though their politics were different, perhaps irreconcilably so. But no more different from where the Establishment and the fascists stood than Katya's and Theo's differences. As Guaril had said almost a decade ago, over breakfast porters at that bohemian café after their ménage a trois that rapturous night before: our blood is red, as our politics, and if the

Nazis ever come to power, both shall be shed on our common stone cell floor . . .

They hiked for the better part of the late September afternoon in the hilly Swiss countryside, the five comrades, old and young, wending their way toward the place where a famous, crazy artist and saloon keeper named Moira Jablonski had a little place off a dusty side road. "Addresses" meant little here, but Quietschend knew the lei of the land, and knew that after so many rises and falls in the earth, they'd find their terminus. And find it they did, as the last rays of the autumnal alpine sun bathed everything in golden crimsons, a god's blazing death in these ancient hills. They came to a small, squat building of gleaming white mud-brick on the side of the dirt road, which they took to be the tavern, their rendezvous point. The sign hanging over the door made them look, and look again.

"El Taqueria del Planta Alpestre?" Theo squinted.

"The Alpine Taco House!" Katya burst out laughing. Not since their days in Spain years ago had they seen Spanish written somewhere so public; and even then, it was the Iberian, the Continental, Castilian, and not the warmer, less formal Latin American, which took precedence. This place looked like a New World hacienda, and seemed the least likely place to be sitting against the Alpine vista behind it.

"This must be the place," Katya concluded, and she led her lover through the low-lintel door.

Inside, it was difficult to tell whether the place was meant to be a tavern, a ski lodge, or an art gallery. Remnants of a dozen cultures, European and otherwise, cluttered the great antechamber and the rooms further in, tall ceilings of mottled cob feigning adobe, with exposed, cedar beams and spinning fans lazily spinning, clouds of smoke that smelt welcomingly of more than just tobacco hanging in a cosy haze amidst the rafters. A running theme amidst the frameless canvases stretched out over the wood and stone were black renderings of bulls. But the reference to Latin America and Iberia that might have been inferred was clouded by the presence of piles of heads, faces of various people the travellers learnt later the artist called her "barnacle people." These faces, painted into every bullish painting over the half dozen in the place, were complimented by the heads of people who hung on the walls in lieu of trophy-kills, Plaster-of-Paris renderings of politicians and infamous, poetaster artists, all defenders of tradition and death. Like the anonymous faces of the Barnacle People, these faces (a young Churchill, a corpse-like Ebert, Marshal Foch, Poincare and Cuno as a double-headed buzzard, Stalin and Lenin and Trotsky as a triple-head, Ramsay-MacDonald, Hoover, Bruning, Braining, Laval, Hindenburg, Mussolini—this last in various poses and ages—and states of drag) looked blankly out to a cold world. But they were all met with warm stares back, the several dozen mountain climbers and hikers and adventurers mingling with the locals, those who looked to one another and the easy, cloudy distance through the great bay windows, and less to the faces on the wall.

The artist responsible for the bulls, the heads, and much of the rest of it, was a tall, thickly- attractive woman of perhaps forty years, her clothes myriad scarves of various patterns and colours, her head nigh shaven to the quick, leaving just a thin grazing of black on her rounded head. She was talking in Romani to a fellow who looked to be Guaril's cousin once or twice removed at the winding bar, then teasing two strapping women in Provençal about their choice of drinks. There was a spread of food on a back table, a smörgåsbord of fish and cheese and herb-drenched vegetables and what appeared a Moroccan hummus, easily a dozen different ethnic foods sharing the same table with no more tensions among them than the dozen nationalities of the patrons of the inn. Theo helped himself to some herring soaked in white-wine vinegar, whilst Katya found a seat for herself at the bar and ordered a shot of cheap American bootleg bourbon.

"A ways from home, eh?" the woman said to her in an Irish-tinted German, smiling winningly as she filled the tall shot glass with the nectar of some southern Yankee province.

"Yeah," Katya said. "'Course, it seems everybody is, here."

"That's true, friend. Nobody's a native here at the hacienda. Most certainly, not me."

"How long've ya had the place?"

"Oh, 'bout four er five years, now. . . . You lookin' to connect with anything . . . *interesting*, during yer stay here in the Alps?"

"I could be. I'm actually looking for some friends."

"Who might they be?"

"Sebastien and Nadia Tovarisch."

"Clever surname. They make it up themselves?"

"Yeah, actually. You speak Russian, too?"

"I speak every language known to man. And quite a few

known to woman. One or two known to dogs . . ."

The agreeable old lass introduced herself at length as Moira Jablonski. The daughter of Polish and Russian parents, raised in Dublin, taught in New York, only to settle here, a stone's throw from Ascona, and the Hill.

"The Hill?"

Katya had heard tell of it from Quietschend, and, too, from Sebastien. The Hill of Truth once stood as a Mecca for crazy communitarians round the turn of the century, just petering out in the last decade or so, though some of the communards were still hanging round here, it was said. Quietschend and Kanalratte and Reinhardt had opted to hike a little on their own. How they would find Katya and Theo again was dubious, at least in Katya's mind; but Quietschend, especially, seemed attune to things in the world, as if he had a compass that could locate any direction, magnetized to find even *people*. He didn't worry.

"Yeah, man," Moira said, pointing through a skylight to the far horizon, "used to be right over there."

Katya looked through the last copper light of the afternoon to a hill in the misty distance. There, in a spot that seemed picturesque in the eerie, stirring way some parts of wild Europe still managed to be, despite thousands of years of cultivation and taming, a hill caught an early alpenglow and almost took her breath away looking at it; almost, for the breath was caught in the shadow of an ugly building which seemed to have recently colonized the place.

"Wow," she said.

"Yeah," Moira agreed. "Not too pretty, huh? Some arschloch bourgeois bought out the commune last year, and built that monstrosity. *Bauhaus*, I believe the kids call it. It's a rich people hotel, built to look like something of 'the People' . . ."

Katya gazed at the unadorned, glassy block darkening the summit of the once communal hill, and understood. She herself had always had a lot of respect for the new things in art and architecture, a lot of hope. But this Bauhaus thing, this seemed indicative of the "bureaucrat" society Theo had theorized about earlier in the last decade: a supposed "workers' architecture," designed not by working people, but *for* them, by the new, intellectual class of benevolent despots. Who would want to live in such an unimaginative, dead thing? She breathed her words aloud, and was surprised to hear them echoed in a familiar voice.

"Who indeed?" the gentle masculine tone lilted beside her.

She turned, to see one of her oldest friends and anarchist comrades. Sebastien, who, marrying Theo's old comrade, had given up his name as she had given up hers, to forge a brand new identity between them. His spectacles were round and made friendlier his friendly eyes, and his black hair was long as a woman's now.

"Sebastien!" she laughed, and embraced him. "How did you sneak in here?!"

"Oh, I've *been* here, comrade. Nadia's round the back, feeding the horses."

"Horses?"

"Yeah. We met up with a pair of 'em, a few years back. It's the only way to travel 'round here . . ."

Horses were an old standby for the Von Rosen household. Katya as Katharina recalled making the acquaintance of more than several over the course of her youth, and forming deep friendships with a few. But those days were long gone. Her bastard parents were in Palestine, they said; they'd probably ground up her old friends into gelatin and glue for the spare pfennigs. Bastards, bastards all.

Katya still knew how to ride a horse well, and she gently, teasingly guided the tenderfoot Theo onto one's back, then mounted it herself, to follow Nadia and Sebastien up the hill to their chalet in the back country outside Ascona. That grim image of the Bauhaus hotel atop the once Truthful Hill became less oppressive and more just something to chuckle at as they passed out of its sight. Many of the communards displaced by that bourgeois hotelier were still hanging around, and a few of them had found their way to the less official, but quite vibrant second-generation commune of the extended family of Sebastien and Nadia, their chalet under the stars. Activists, wanted by various governments in Europe—especially Fascist Italy, which surrounded the canton the chalet stood in on three sides—passed through here looking for asylum. Literati, too, of the rebel kind, found refuge under Sebastien and Nadia's roof— staying together in a loose, international confederation called the Guild of Libertarian Bibliophiles, just formed in 1929, for which the chalet was a sometime meeting place.

One particular couple spanned both of these categories, activist and literati, and had been founding members of the Guild. They were as exciting and gentle as any artist-terrorists could be, as the travellers spent their first night at the place. They'd stay for the next weeks at the Tovarisch Chalet, as the generous autumn gave way to the mildest of winters, keeping Katya and her Theo and their young friends company for almost the entirety of their stay.

"Call me Erich," smiled the bearded, bespectacled fellow to Katya as the moon rose over the Alpine horizon that first evening.

"Is that your *real* name?" Katya flirted with him, her bottle of old Kentucky moonshine bourbon hanging from careless fingers on the veranda. "I've always had a *particular* fondness for fellows with that name."

"Oh, it's one of my many," he smiled back. Then, he put his hand on the arm of an older woman beside him. "And this is my Zenzl."

"Hello," smiled the pretty lady to Katya. It seemed a little formal, the older man's taking the older woman's arm. Time would tell it wasn't possession, surely not ownership that motivated that "my" in *my Zenzl*. Everyone in the chalet would play together, and well, over the next weeks. But before there was such trust, there had to be talk, honest and loving, in the privacy of each partnership. Erich and Zenzl's talk had not yet happened, at least concerning this new, young, beautiful woman who teased the elder Erich so invitingly. Until that talk could be had, Erich gallantly distanced his smile from the young woman's admiring eyes, and squeezed his partner's arm.

Theo was standing some yards away from the house with Quietschend, who had come upon them out of some bushes near the sloping roadside, having tracked them all as they made their way through the Alpine foothills as if by a sixth sense. He'd jumped out at them, saying **"BOOOO-MSEN!!!"** with Reinhardt right behind—startling Katya and Theo and Sebastien and Nadia, but curiously, not their horses. Theo and Quietschend were looking now onto his mother's land, which neighboured the little property of Sebastien and Nadia as if by some divinely-hinting coincidence.

"You're right, man," Theo was telling him. "This place is . . . quite the place."

They looked down into a valley where people were sparring, fighting, playing mock-deadly games of hide and seek amidst the palms and scrub brush. A group had grabbed the flag—from here, in the moonlight, Theo couldn't tell whether it was the black flag or the red one—and were taking it across a stream to a hiding place in the rocks. Further on, in an open field which at this time of night and year was becoming misty, so the figures seemed spectral, perhaps twenty people were taking aim at as many targets, locking and loading and pumping the bull's eyes full of lead.

Quietschend smiled.

"I know, chum," he said. "I know."

Theo turned to the chalet. Katya was on the veranda, looking happier and sexier than she had in years, her head resting on Nadia's shoulder as the two women leaned on a far railing. Sebastien was discussing logistics with Reinhardt and some older folks on the steps, including a very striking man with a dark beard and moustache, short but thickly wild hair, and spectacles which caught the glint of the bonfire some others were building in front of the house.

"Where's Kanalratte?" Theo asked. "I didn't see sie when you jumped out at us back there."

"Oh, sie'll be along, chum. I think sie's the one who grabbed the flag . . ."

They ate dinner al fresco in the great sward in front of the chalet, strawberries and chocolate and smuggled Italian champagne. Sebastien bonded with Theo as an old comrade, no matter that they'd once not been, offering now shared sympathies for the dismal state of Europe and the co-optation of radicalism by the commies. The fellow with the beard sat across a blanket, his head in the lap of his wife, the pretty, older woman everybody called Zenzl, letting her feed him strawberries and drams of Prosecco between tender kisses. Kanalratte had returned with a host of young comrades, all beaten and dirty and laughing tough, satisfied laughs. They were ready, sie said. Sie wanted to storm the Reichstag right now, or invade Italy and succeed in killing the bloody Duce where three people in the last year had failed—all with an army too young to conscript. The dark-bearded fellow urged caution.

"There'll be time for that," he smiled. "Not to worry, comrades."

His name was Erich Mühsam, though he'd been known by many other names over his history as an anarchist. He regaled them with stories over the next hours, as they curled together on the hill of the chalet in the hours after their dinner, disdaining the indoors and cosiness of the hearth to drink strong Irish whiskey round their fire pit in the earth. Erich spoke of his youthful rebelliousness, beatings from a Prussian boarding school and an awful father, and a scandal he'd caused in the school with some youthful writings in an underground newspaper he'd helped put together, exposing the corruption of the headmasters. "Got me kicked soundly out of that hell-hole," he laughed, "which is a primary reason I did it . . ." He spoke of that wondrous spring of '19 in Bavaria, when he and his comrades Ernst Toller and Gustav Landauer and many, many others had forced the thick-headed moribund aristocrat Ludwig from the throne and declared Bavaria an independent, soviet republic—the best birthday present he ever had.

"The doctrinaire '-ists' ruined it, though," he reminisced. "You know, friends: commun-ists, social-ists, even some anarch-ists. Too into their theories to recognize—and *respect*—the spontaneity of the regular working people. Fuck theor-ists, friends! To hell with art-ists and drama-tists, too!"

"Oh, Erich, dear," smiled Zenzl, "you do drive a hard line, don't you now?"

"I'm serious, love!"

"You always are."

"Come, dear-heart. You know exactly what I'm saying. And you know it's *sense*."

"Oh, I'm not faulting your logic, *Herr* Mühsam. Just your brazenness."

"Oh! My vigour bothers you, then!"

"No, dear-heart. Just your *stridency*. You're very, very *loud*, mein herr."

"Ah!—*ah*. Ah, yes. You're right," he smiled. "When Zenzl pronounces, it's worth its weight in diamonds."

"What does breath actually weigh, though?" Quietschend challenged.

"Oh, dear squeaky! That fully depends on where it's aimed."

Erich then sprung up and ran off.

"Where's he going?" Theo asked.

Zenzl just smiled and shrugged.

Sebastien came out to the fire with Reinhardt and Kanalratte beside him. They were wearing overcoats, very heavy, even for the suddenly chill alpine night. Kanalratte laughed as everyone looked to them.

"Well?" sie asked. "What d'ya think?"

"About what?" Katya asked.

"About *us*," Reinhardt directed, lifting his arms, spinning in place.

"You look quite fetching," laughed Theo, "both of you."

"Do we look," Kanalratte smirked—"unusual?"

"A bit overdressed," said Zenzl.

"Fashionable, though," Nadia added.

"Passable?" Reinhardt pressed. "I mean, as on a train?"

"You need hats," Quietschend said emphatically. "Yes, definitely hats."

Kanalratte smiled to Sebastien.

"Hats," Sebastien said, "can be arranged. . . . But, what *else?*"

Everyone looked blankly at the young pair.

"I wove these threads special," Sebastien said, as if playing one of those guessing games they would entertain each other with on rainy nights over the next weeks by the hearth, when al fresco dining on the hill would prove impracticable. "Do you—*admire* my designs?"

Before anyone could answer, Sebastien smiled to his friends.

"Why don't you two show them the coup de gras?"

Kanalratte and Reinhardt opened their overcoats, and pointed to the almost imperceptible wires lining the insides, disappearing into the sleeves, leading straight down into the lower pockets.

The observers still drew a blank.

"You know," Sebastien said dreamily, "the history of our hypocritical European custom—the *handshake?*"

"No," Zenzl laughed, "but I think you're about to tell us."

"Indeed. They say it came from the era of feudalism, when travellers in the wilds and fens between towns met on the road. They used their right hands—*thus*—to make sure neither of the brutes would draw a sword on the other. Now, of course, the handshake is the symbol of masculine familiarity. It is used to seal contracts, business deals, the fates of nations. But how far have we really come??"

Before anyone could speculate what the queer fellow meant, Kanalratte and Reinhardt were shaking hands, dramatically, over and over. As they did so, their bulky sleeves touched—and *sealed together.* Then, as the buttons touched, the sound of a spring catching went off in both their overcoats. Something small dropped down to the ground.

"Then we all run!"

Kanalratte turned round and ran back, as did Reinhardt, guffawing as they ran to separate sides of the chalet. Sebastien stepped aside, as a soft, sharp hissing sounded amidst them. The little thing on the ground, invisible in the darkness for its small size and black colour, began tinging the Mozart theme from *The Magic Flute* that signalled Emil Jannings' fall to Marlene Dietrich in the first talkie in Germany.

Sebastien picked it up, and showed them the little clockwork thing. It was round and black, somewhere between a compass and a wristwatch in size. It buzzed a little in his hands. Then, as the little Papageno ditty ended, he threw it down into the valley. A great spark like ball lightning flashed long before it hit the ground.

"It doesn't have to sing, of course," he smiled to the disbelieving little crowd of his friends. "I just put that there to—"

"—To show off," Nadia smiled, and smiling, Sebastien conceded the point.

"Wow!" Katya exclaimed. "But, surely, your little magic trick wouldn't damage that much."

"That," Sebastien smiled, "is where the coats come in. Guys! If you would!!"

Kanalratte and Reinhardt returned, laughing at some private joke between them. They took off their coats, and lay them on the ground for their friends' inspection. Examining the lining, they found a quantity of gunpowder and nitroglycerin in long, thin tubes sewn in, a dozen tubes if one.

"Of course," Sebastien explained with pride, "that little spark would have a far greater impact if, after our two friends met and shook, one or both of them would take off their coats—as, say, one does when one enters a cabin in a second or first class compartment of a train car."

"Why do they have to shake hands?"

"Oh, that's just for drama," laughed Erich, returning, a new bottle in his arm, "*nicht wahr, Kameraden*?"

"Yes," Sebastien said with a delicious flourish. "A dramatic effect. You could also just cross your own arms, if alone. Or cross your legs. Or, many other things, I suppose."

"Wouldn't you end up blowing yourself up, too?" Katya demanded suddenly.

"I can set the magnetized detonator for up to an hour after the initial 'kiss.' But, of course, you'd probably not need that much time."

"So, it's the magnets that do it?" Theo asked.

"Yes. My own invention, I'm . . . proud to say."

"My Vati helped," Quietschend said, "though, he never knew he helped. . . . There's advantages to interning in the family lab."

Magnets, of course, had been Sebastien's passion for years, Theo and Katya recalled. From the first conversations Theodor had with him, the Swiss eccentric had been promoting the many and varied uses of magnets, advocating their use in everything from psychic and physical health to alternative sources of electrical power. Wilhelm Reich came up, as he had already that night and would again over the next nights, his concept of the *orgonne*, which again Sebastien explained, and Nadia swore by (though neither could really explain it coherently). There was energy laden in everything alive, from the force of the wind to the dizzy potency of orgasm; and magnets tapped into this power like nothing else. So simple, they were, so apparently safe and innocuous. And in that, deceptive.

Quietschend was talking about something his physicist father had been going on about since he was a small boy in the Komagome neighbourhood of Tokyo, in the shadow of the first laboratory building of the RIKEN complex there—something the old man wanted to build. An accelerator of particles, molecules, atoms, and even smaller quanta. The whole thing would be driven by magnets. Sebastien and Quietschend debated quantum mechanics for the next half hour, then, as Erich pontificated about the irrelevance of Napoleon and Zenzl teased him for a prig. Theo laid his head on Katya's lap, as she lay in the arms of Nadia. They dreamt together, aloud, of propaganda of the deed. So much theorizing, they theorized together, had to do with avoiding action, putting it off, getting other people to do it. In the end, they agreed, it wasn't about what you thought, what you said, what you knew. It was about what you *did*. And, one action, even something as small as sneaking a good fuck in a second class compartment of a speeding train, could move mountains . . .

Erich's plays had been celebrated over the years, but had been performed only erratically and occasionally. His latest one, *All Hang!*, had never been officially put on anywhere. Though he made no money from it, and none but the small crowd round them would appreciate it, the wonderful play calling for Revolution as the only cure for the plague of Nazism was acted out in Sebastien's and Nadia's chalet, half according to Erich's dog-eared script, half improvised by the actors on his theme. Kanalratte and Reinhardt distinguished themselves in starring roles, and even Theo and Katya, who had never acted before in their lives, injected an element of spontaneity into the production: Theo recalled speeches he'd heard Karl Liebknecht make when he was barely more than a child, in the first days of the German Revolution, mingling them with the words of his father, Wilhelm, told to him by his own father, years and years before; and Katya played a balalaika and sang an old highwayman's lament, a lullaby Guaril had sung to her during a depression she'd mired in nearly a decade ago, something she'd sung to herself to regain her mind in her drug hangovers following the weeks of dreamless slumber in her first winter in the sanatorium. The father's words and the lover's song weren't part of the script, of course, but Erich welcomed them, and they provided a fine intermezzo when they put the play on in an informal, unofficial performance at the tavern where they'd first met up in in Ascona, run by the tough, pretty internationalist bartender Moira. Erich had long thought pubs and cabarets were no place to put on serious, political plays; but with Zenzl teasing him again for a prig, and the general joy of the crowd the old anarchist playwright found himself in, Erich Mühsam conceded the attraction of putting on his play in such a setting as the Alpine Taqueria, even though no one would remember it the next morning.

Nobody besides a score of drunken patrons would ever see *All Hang!* in Erich's lifetime, nor in the lifetimes of any of the actors who put it on in that smoky, cosy Alpine tavern. No one would know what the play was, what it meant, most all the copies of it burnt in an offering to the Nazi Gods of Ignorance in the coming years. But, like all the things which transpired in this era which would not last the night, elements of it, like a half-remembered dream, would haunt future eras, sowing the seeds of new phantoms in the nocturnes to follow the long, desiccating Nazi Dawn.

There were still a few more hours of the Night left, though. Before they all departed from one another's company forever, in the last days of 1931, each of them would have the chance to share a goodnight kiss. The night after their performance at the Alpine Taqueria, people had fallen into each other and taken each other to the various beds of the chalet. Erich was left nursing a bottle and old memories in the hall before the great hearth, nestling into an armchair. Katya found him, and sat close to him, nursing him on tales of her youthful rebellion, and opening herself up to what tales of older rebellions he might fill her with. She suckled on his wisdom a long while, as they shared the bottle of warm Kirschwasser. She glanced at him, over and over as they talked. He kept staring into the fire.

"Have you been with Zenzl a long time, Erich?"

He sighed softly.

"We've been married since 1915. Though we've known each other longer."

"Why did you marry?"

"Ah, well. It was a different time, then, before the War ended. Neither Zenzl or I believed in marriage, *per se*. But there were . . . reasons . . ."

Katharina looked to the older man's face, the shadows the fire made on it, and tried to read his thoughts. But he'd a lifetime of thoughts hidden beneath that wild beard, those spectacles, those leathery wrinkles. Years of jail-time, of persecution and hiding, of fights on the barricades and lonely privation, trying to make a living in the cabaret and by his plays—none of which ever shirked from telling the truth—a truth that many people still did not want to hear. At thirty years, just turned, she was as a little girl in his wizened presence; he'd reached thirty when she was but a girl of six. He'd long practised the arts of not revealing his thoughts, his soul, so long he'd probably learnt how not to reveal them even to himself.

"I was just thirteen for most of 1915," she laughed, pulling out of the awkward silence. He smiled, and recalled with sympathy and respect the story she'd told him on her first night, of the involuntary incarceration she'd suffered when her analyst died by his own hand, how she'd languished in that sanatorium till she'd run away a year and a half later and gotten together with her great aunt in Switzerland.

He'd been listening to her, then . . .

"You're both so beautiful together," she said of Erich and Zenzl. "I can understand why you married each other. If Theo and I believed in it, we might well have done it, too."

"Yes, well, I think times are changing," he mused, "toward *our* way, in some wise. The freer, anarchic way. It is much more possible, now, to go without that marriage license—let alone some church or rabbinical ceremony, to allow y'all to fuck. You're a great generation, Katya—as is the one coming up now, after you. It gives an old man hope."

She looked at him sharply, and smiled a sly smile.

"You ain't so old," she said.

He laughed deeply.

"Ah, but I am! Let's not ignore what's obvious between us, kitten—this lifetime that lives in the years between us. Those years, their *energies,* could quicken us both, I think."

They both found themselves smiling, sharing a look across the parlour. The look lasted a long time. But then, his thoughts went back behind his eyes, lost again to Katharina. He seemed a man who was weighing all the years of his life, counting them, and realizing with a certain fearfulness, yet struggling for a grim resignation—the best pose he could muster—that there were very few of them left. He took a long swallow of the Kirschwasser.

"I do worry about my Zenzl. She's a dedicated soul—stronger than I—and I flatter myself to think myself strong. I see hard years ahead of us. But especially for her. In the dawn to come, it might be good to—to *sleep in*—to sleep *forever,* and not awaken for that day. It's not hard for me to contemplate such laziness—spiritual, following the physical. I've spent half a century in this lifetime already, kitten—and already a few years more. But Zenzl is younger than I. She, I fear, will go on. And what kind of world have I left her with, eh . . . ?"

Katya drew herself towards him, knelt by his armchair, and kissed his hand.

"You're so brave, so good, Erich," she said softly. "If only more or our race were as brave and good."

"Ah! If more of our race, Katya—more of us hairless apes—were 'brave' and 'good' like me—Ah! The world might be a very tragic world indeed! Zenzl is right about me, you know. I *am* a prig. No, my girl, I *am!* A prig, and worse, I fear . . . a *snob.* I'm still chewing over our decision to show *All Hang!* at that hacienda last night. It seems almost a—a sacrilege, to mix one kind of cabaret with another." He laughed, shaking his head at the fire. "I've always been ambivalent about cabaret. On the one hand, I've made my living by it, in the small way that I've made my living—yet, on the other hand, I've always been uncomfortable with the—the lack of *seriousness* that you often find there. It's like the arts of dance, and film; so often you find gems there, really wonderful works—that can *live,* you know? In the minds of people, eh? That can inspire them to take *action.* But those gems are so often buried in mountains of slag."

"Do you like modern dance, Erich?"

"Yes, some of it. I was always fascinated by the prevalence of the naked dances, the whole culture of nudity—a barrier-breaking, and often revolutionary thing—yet infected, too, with the most horrible, 'race-purity' eugenics nonsense on the one hand, and the most prurient motivations, on the other. I always admired the idealism of such people as Ida Herion, and Ernst Schertel—"

"Oh, I *love* Ernst Schertel! I've always loved his choreography—and his photography, too! I actually met him a few times, years ago. Carried a torch for him, a little, back then, I'm both embarrassed *and* proud, to admit."

"Yes, as I say, I admired his idealism; though not always his actual practice. His use of such *young* dancers, to do the kinds of dances he wanted to make—those strange, dark orgies of choreography . . . I was always more a fan of Mary Wigman—she studied under an old acquaintance of mine, Rudolf Laban, at the old Hill of Truth, not far from this chalet, during the War, you know."

"I didn't know that."

"Ah, yes. A talent she had—still has, surely. One of the finest dancers and choreographers of our time. She always impressed me. . . . But then, such a person is *supposed to* impress one—isn't it true, kitten? Again—ah, again I play the snob . . . You know, I once wrote a scathing review of Anita Berber's dancing. A fine talent she had. If it weren't for the pills and the booze, she might still be dancing with us."

"And the *sex,*" Katya said, gazing up with a knowing, naughty grin from where she knelt.

"Ah. Ah, no. I've no problem with *that.* That was one of the few things she did right. Fucking never hurt anyone. It's the sicknesses they put in the waters, in the humours . . ."

Again his face set against the fire. She wanted to loosen the muscles of that face, to crack that ponderous façade. Her heart quickened, and she heard her breath rasp beneath his words.

"You know what happened, kitten? That poor, wounded darling wrote me, and *begged* me to 'reconsider' my review. Not for fame, or money—no, nothing so trite. The review was already published, the damage done. It was because—because—"

He looked down at her, and tried to smile. In the end, though, he gave up on it, and said, "Because she really wanted my respect. She wanted me to understand her. To appreciate her, alongside someone like Wigman. Wigman's dances have always proceeded from her writing—notebooks, strewn with notes, furiously scribbled—and from there, she makes her dances. Ah, perhaps that's why I've admired her better. She's like me in that regard: she *plans.* But that poor, wounded darling, that misunderstood icon, Anita; her planning always proceeded from the dance, her poetry, her pictures—but then, it'd go back *into* the dance—a more *real* art-form—the poetry, the photographs and sketches *entwined* with the action—the body and the mind as *one.* Even when she failed to achieve her best performances, as the one I reviewed that time—even then, she had such a . . . *sincerity.* And when I wrote my—my *cruelty* towards her—she actually *apologized*—to **me!** For failing . . . She even told me she'd 'try better' . . . Ah, sometimes, kitten, you have more power than you realize, even when you strive against the urge to power with every breath of your being . . . and, you—*hurt* people . . . hurt those you never, never meant to . . . *Ahhhh* . . ."

What strange thoughts were churning beneath that iconic visage? A lifetime's worth of memories and regrets. Katya wanted to throw herself at him—to offer herself to him any way she could!

But, *how?*

She looked up at him, caught his eye. He tried to smile, and so did she. But in the end, they just stared, as if each trying to understand the strange creature looking at him, at her. Without another word, she loosened her shawl, and then the folds of the diaphanous blouse beneath it—both ten years behind the times now, out-of-fashion, verging on old-fashioned. She rubbed her forward-snapping brassiere against the clasps of his boots, and unsnapped it—an old trick she'd learned as a boot-girl with Johanna at her side in the Wittenberg Platz. She let the brassiere fall with the rest.

His eyes did not move from hers. They were dark, and deep, and they went on forever. She was offering her body, but he was not looking at her body. He wanted something more, something harder to give.

She hugged his legs, and opened hers round them, determined to give him everything—all he wanted, and all he did not yet know he wanted—inviting him to go inside and *take* it. He sighed, deep, low, with a fluttering at the edges. The first crack in the façade.

She rubbed her face against his knees, his thighs, his middle. She licked at his tweed trousers, far from just out of fashion, thoroughly ancient now, a relic of the last century. Could she not see the little worn seams, the little tears, that Zenzl had darned?

She wanted that role suddenly, as she rubbed and danced below him. To sit beside the older woman, and minister to her, helping her minister to him. She'd never displace Zenzl as the love of his life. She did not want to. But she longed to be a lesser light beside her, a Morningstar beside her Sunlight over Erich's Earth.

He smelled of the earth. Not the smell of dirt, or rottenness—but the clean, mineral smell of the mountain streams, of how she imagined the smell of the mountains themselves. A Giant he was, in the eldest, Wagnerian sense—in the best sense of that sense. A mythic, chthonic figure.

What strange thoughts filled her now! As she caressed his outer thighs with her strong, soft arms, and kissed his lower parts in homage, as she'd done for money as well as pleasure so many hundreds of times before, she was embarrassed by these thoughts. But she clung to them anyway, swallowing the embarrassment and letting it redden her dusky eggshell skin, keeping it in her head and in her gut, to burn there, in painful pleasure. A lesser wife, she could be to this Prince Among Men. A slave-girl—an odalisque in this great man's harem—a captured nymph in the Hall of the Mountain King. A blind, zealous *follower* . . .

She laughed at her thoughts, disdaining his breathy, awkward offer of more Kirschwasser before he clumsily corked it for the night and let it fall to the floor beside them; like him, she'd had more than enough—her thoughts swimming with her sensations, feeling small, and delighted in that, on her knees at the feet of this man who had almost single-handedly made history. Such thoughts as she was revelling in would be an insult to the great man, a man who was great because he was not, because he eschewed greatness, had pledged his life to its abolition. Yet, her sexuality was not her politics, but a mummery. A symbol, a sigil, an allegory of that which she opposed, even feared. To play with those tropes was to deny their real power. Old Erich she made a Pharaoh, a King upon his throne. She could never worship him this way if he didn't himself so hate the pharaohs and the kings.

She breathed a prayer to her godless God, when she'd reached the innermost part of His raiment, beseeching Him to allow her to continue her homage with a soft and prayerful look up at him, her mouth open as if to speak, her lips moist with anticipation. He granted her plea with a gentle stroke of her cheek and a smoothing of her hair.

She'd touched her lips to every darned rip and frayed seam of his tweed trousers, and now touched the rip that had been purposefully placed there. She licked the zip open, then fluttered her tongue into the cunt-like crack till a part of him arose to greet her there.

She closed her lips in a deep purr round the perfect circle of his cock-head, welcoming with smooth, strong strokes of her soft hands his sliding further in. Again a sigh, almost of astonishment, and then another, longer sigh, ringing like the cathedral bells had rung on his forty-first birthday in Bavaria, above her bobbing head.

She closed tight around him, her breasts sharp soft stroking his woollen, raspy trousers, delighting in the burns of weft and warp upon her flesh. All of him beneath his navel was hers now, and his elder bones quickened and danced across her young girl's tongue, the old man's whole universe in those long, delicious instants.

He stroked her black hair furiously, pulling at bunches of it behind her nape and driving himself into her. She swallowed her breath and all he gave her, his earthy scents mingling with the sharpness of her own sweat breaking on her breast and neck as she let the rhythm of sucking and swallowing take over her consciousness and drown it in blacknesses and lights and *wanting*. A young man he was, a boy now, a passion that pulled down decades of practised propriety like the gates of a Winter Palace, this moment in history when quantity sublates into quality and all things boil over.

Salt, like earth, and fecund fungal tastes flooded Katya's throat as she surrendered to the channelling of power from his deepest heart into hers. She kept her lips and tongue swirling round him till he softened, till he gently tugged her hair away.

She looked up to him and smiled, a coy girl who knew her daddy better than he knew himself. He gazed at her, a long, delirious, grateful minute from on high. Then, he avalanched down from the chair, tossing his spectacles aside and rending his shirt, buttons flying off—and pushed her back on the floor on the raw rock extension of the hearthstone, softened by a thick Afghan kilim. He kissed his own cum from her lips as she giggled in triumph, then dove into her breasts and sucked and bit them with a young man's vigour, a boy's hunger. He devoured her, down her belly to her silken skirt which he tore in twain so he might feast upon the black curls and red flesh of her pulsing, glistening pussy, offering her his hungry homage to match her own. She stroked his wild hair, tossing his curls and playing with them, tightening her grip as shivers danced though every inch of her softly screaming flesh. She came and came, tightening her thighs against his furry face till she thought she'd drown him—till she'd almost drowned herself. And he came again, drunk with her hot smells and burning tastes and the raging joy of the gift they gave each other—groaning hot into her cunt so its sound sang up her spine, almost loud enough to drown in her own ears her own deep contralto roaring.

They curled together and slept a long while as the fire beside them died down to embers. She awoke in the night, with the older man's curly head on her breast, and stretched lazily against his warm, furry curves in perfect bliss. Her eyes panned across the room to the archway leading toward the inner chambers of the chalet. Zenzl was standing there, and seemed to have been standing there for a long while, gazing at her in silence. Sebastien and Theo were in each of her arms, their eyes half-moon, Theo's head nestling into her grey shoulder.

All three of them were softly smiling . . .

Chapter 22

The next year flew by, as time flows when happy times are upon you. Katya and Theo watched as their Edelweiss Pirate friends grew older, feeling uncannily like parents, or rather, like an aunt and an uncle, to the brave, crazy children coming into a revolutionary maturity, defying the adult world round them. Kanalratte remained of a consciously dubious gender, refusing the enticements of the straight world to conform with one or another aspect of *ihre Faktizitat,* ihre facticity. Sie did not care to define selbst, and with *ihre Furchtlosigkeit und Körperiche tűchtigkeit,* ihre fearlessness and physical prowess, not even the Brownshirts could force sie to choose. It was freer this way, sie said, and Theo and Katya, no strangers to the great wealth of gender inversion that had marked their generation, only blest the young androgyne's attitude. Reinhardt and Quietschend continued to be their friends, too, as well as dozens of other wayward youth of the nascent Edelweiss Pirates, whose ranks grew with every passing season. The Hitler Youth, and the girls' auxiliary to that miserable band, continued to alienate people, even as their ranks swelled with happy campers and bicyclists, still enamoured with the healthy, bucolic pursuits that had defined those organizations since their inception. The cult of the body, the cult of health, was a very enticing and entrancing fetish in the sickly world of declining Berlin, and the young people who flocked to those organizations, and the activities round them, celebrated their fitness for the new, dawning world as some divine birthright. Kanalratte, disdaining alcohol and tobacco and a hundred other vices sie considered stupid, pointless invasions of the adult world into *ihre Körper,* ihre body, embraced health in those seasons, too; not for the typical worship the world round sie mired in—the quest for the "perfect, Aryan superman"—but rather for the chance health would give sie for giving hell to the powers that be. Sie did not want to die—at least, not until sie could do something substantive, something *important* with *ihr Leben.* Sie didn't see living much past thirty, or even twenty; but sie'd be damned if sie died a corrupted death of cigarettes and venereal diseases and beer. Sie would die when sie wanted to, for ihre own reasons, *ihre eigenen Gründe* —soon perhaps, but only on ihre own terms. And *irhe Kameraden Edelweißpiraten* embraced healthy living for exactly the same reasons.

Katya delighted in cooking for these young people,

mulligan stews she made of all the fare the kids found or stole over the day. She delighted in housing them, too, keeping them safe and warm in the bitter gales of the world, and she went out of her way to maintain the second incarnation of the slum salon with these young people as the primary members of the wide circle. Theo chatted with them all, talking of things which would continue to affect the world long after he himself was dead, issues of class and civilisation, racism and war. But in the forward-thinking ethos of the salon, such things paled into the passé. The kids who hung around now were not interested in theory, but in *action*. They did not concern themselves with art, or philosophy, or any other cultural middlemen in their struggle to be free and alive. They saw the world's progress to its inexorable end as an opportunity to make something crazy and beautiful in the ruins, and the ruins were all around them right *now*. Weimar would fade, they all knew; what came after was of little concern, for they would not live beyond it. These young, vibrant people only wanted to go out with a resounding, and significant, bang.

"Fuck T.S. Eliot," spat the pretty, Ashkenazi girl named Naomi they'd met a year ago in the Underground mouse hole of the Pirates, after a performance in one of the sleazier *Nachtlokal* cabarets where she'd been dancing lately, enticing old bourgeois to spend their marks on her to give them a little tease at intimacy, before they fell into drunken stupor on the floors of the abandoned flats she'd take them to. Then she'd steal the rest of their money, leaving them broke and bitterly hungover in the cold, grey dawns alone. Naomi, with her proud Star of David round her neck, amidst all her lace and garters and enticing accoutrements of sex-crazy, sex-starved Berlin, could have been a younger sister to that Chonte prostitute who, years before, had fought beside Katya and Theo and Theo's old comrade, Klaus, when they'd ambushed that Nazi meeting after drinking all night at the old Black Tie. But Naomi was from east of Lublin, east of Poland, from that lost land of Russia where her uncle had killed three czarist officers in 1915 in retaliation for a pogrom that had claimed her parents' lives, and had to flee westward with the newborn and two of her sisters here to Deutschland. Naomi was beautiful and angry, dark-haired and curvy and bespectacled, and danced this anger into every bend of her knees, arms, and hips. It drove the old bourgeois wild; but she was more into getting them drunk and ripping them off than servicing them in any real way. Katya and Theo liked her, as all the young Pirates, bringing her round to stay for days or weeks at a time in their slum salon.

Naomi began to bring a new boy around toward the end of 1932, a fellow named "Dempsey," after the American boxer Jack Dempsey. An unemployed-activist, drifter, and occasional bricklayer from Holland, he fit well into the Pirates' scene even though he was a little older than most of them in his early twenties. His parents had been divorced, then both died before he'd reached fifteen years of age. Dempsey was thus an orphan and a vagabond for years before he connected with the slum salon, which put him in good company. He'd joined the Dutch Communist Party in '30 or '31, but soon left it, though he was still a communist in theory and practice, something that caused more than one heated debate between him and Naomi, who was as much an anarchist as Katya or Theo, though not so much because of what she'd read as what she'd lived and seen. Neither Naomi nor Dempsey, nor most everyone else in the scene had as much use for "theories" as those of Theo's and Katya's generation. The greatest theories were already out there, *had been* out there—and the world had gone on in its fucked up way despite it all.

Dempsey was a good fellow, but a bit determined to be the hero. He told everyone that he'd been blinded in one eye with lye at the Tielmann factory in Leiden, Holland, and then during a strike that broke out there, he'd tried to claim sole responsibility for it to the management, to keep the heat off all his comrades. Dempsey wanted to be a martyr, it seemed. But such mild insanity was not uncommon in the circle of the slum salon, now or in the past, and further, Katya more than once actually phrased the sentiment that, if more people in the populace had such complexes of martyrdom, and were willing to actually *do* something about it—the world might not be the horrible place it was today.

Katya began talking in earnest on this tangent. Action was the only thing left for them, she said, more urgent, more real than what was said or sung or written about. One by one, the great magazines and papers that had defined the radical here in Berlin were folding. *Der Sturm* petered out that year, and a lot of the queer papers began printing less and less often, too. The last issues of *Die Freundin* stopped putting pictures of naked, beautiful lesbians on their covers, almost as if trying to slip under the censors which had halted its publication in 1926 under the Protection of Youth From Obscene Publications Act—something from which the Girlfriend's magazine never really recovered. There was something desperate in the blank covers, a concession to defeatism even before final defeat. And *Die Aktion*, the far-left paper that was amongst the only friendly ones to Theo and Katya and Guaril back in the day, published just once in the whole year of 1930, and but twice in 1931. Katya, who had met its publisher Franz Pfemfert years ago when the magazine was going strong, and knew well his wife, Alexandra, to whom Katya had given a whole series of articles for the art magazine she published with Franz, came to their long-time flat at the end of the Nassauische Straße, the fourth floor of number 17, in Wilmersdorf, to ask what was up. Alexandra was nowhere to be found, evidently spending most of her time lately travelling further and further out from Berlin and their old haunts, drumming up what she could to support Franz and herself. Franz was frittering away the afternoon at his desk, trying to write something, but mostly just rolling endless cigarettes on a machine. "I've got great plans, Katharina," he assured in gusts of frenetic smoke, his hand pushing back his back-slicked hair—"They won't beat us yet!" But no further issues came from there that year, and when Katya visited again a month or two later, the flats were empty, a notice of eviction lying in the dust in the hall outside.

As 1932 closed in on 1933, and the Communists peaked in the polls, then began to lose their following amongst the German people to the Nazis, Katya lifted herself with gruelling effort out of many a spell of melancholia—the fire of action her only steady light. Propaganda of the Deed became the sole thing she was holding out for. Kanalratte, and Reinhardt, and Quietschend, and Naomi and Dempsey and dozens of others amongst the Pirates, that queer mix of the anarchist and the communist and the simply riled up young people of a moribund Weimar, began making connections between the different cities where their activisms and their lifestyles converged into some last, defiant stand against the government and against the fascists that seemed destined to inherit it. People began talking seriously of making a strike against these enemy, reactionary forces. People began talking of burning down the edifices of power, whether the "masses" would follow the riled, fed up vanguard into rebellion or not.

Theo struggled with paranoia that seemed of another world from the terrible, paranoid world Germany was becoming. He'd had the uncanny feeling of being followed for many months, to the point where he didn't want to go out of the flat even for a loaf of bread or a bottle of beer. He heard the conversations of passers-by on the street signalling and signing to him of a narrative he would not tell Katya or any of his friends the details of; he did not even seem particularly capable of facing these details himself. But the narrative was heavy on him towards the end of 1932, making him question everything, making him suspect everything and everyone. His madness fell sickly in step with the madness of the world round him. And whilst his Katya praised him for his courage, and even contemplated some art or poetry that could reflect the connections between the world outside and the world within him, and perhaps bridge the two in some kind of healing—she could not hope to understand the tangles of his mad world, and could do little in the end but offer her desperate, ignorant sympathy.

One night, coming home from a show where Naomi had done her burlesque to the horrid cheers of a hundred ugly men and women of decadent Berlin, Theo was walking up the stairs to his and Katya's apartment, and came face to face with a man that seemed a figure from a nightmare. Tall, pale, laughing maniacally, with a beard of grizzled white all the way down his chest, barefoot in ragged pyjamas he'd seemed to have worn for years without changing them, Theodor saw the man who'd been laughing in the apartment below them for a whole decade. A lonely man. Disfigured by time, and untold anxieties. The man stood there, in Theo's way, on the landing before the third floor, and home.

"Excuse me, mein herr," Theo said, bowing slightly, "but, would you mind moving aside?"

"You know me," the man said.

Theo looked to him quizzically.

"Do I, sir?"

"Yes, you do. And, I know *you.*"

Theo looked at him, laughing nervously.

"Do you now?"

"Yes, boy. I have known you for ten thousand years. And, you have known me. Yet, we have never before this night spoken a word to one another."

"That's true, sir."

The old man laughed, coughing and sputtering and wheezing.

"I have lived in this tenement since it was erected, young man. And the foundations of this building were laid when Deutschland was still a pagan country, when Berlin was Polabian swamp! And you've been traipsing up and down these steps all this time. And you never bothered to knock at my door, and ask me how I was."

"I'm . . . sorry, sir. I never thought—"

"Yeah, *that's* the truth! You never, *ever* thought!!"

Possessed by a desire to ameliorate, to welcome, and tipsy with more than his share of beer at Naomi's cabaret, Theodor stepped forward and offered his hand to the strange old man.

"Theo's my name, sir," he said. "What's yours?"

The man put a limp, cold hand in Theo's, and said, "My name is 'Sanity.'"

"Eh?"

"My name, my son, is Sanity. And I shall die tomorrow. We are strangers, you and I. And nothing can change that, now. I've been sitting in my little, dirty flat these past ten years, laughing, weeping. But, tonight shall be my last night on this earth, little boy. What will you say of me?"

"Pardon, sir?"

"What will you *say* of me, boy?! When I am **gone?!**"

Theodor looked at him, speechless. He really just wanted to get past the figure now, and go to his bed, and sleep after his long night on the town. Katya would be waiting, perhaps with some pretty boy or pretty girl of the Edelweiss Pirates, to comfort them in the night with some illicit, beautiful gift of themselves. Theo wanted to go home.

"I'm sorry," he said, "that we never knew each other, *alter.*"

"Perhaps—in another life??"

Theo smiled at the maniac smile.

"Yes, perhaps."

"I'm leaving, boy! Sanity is leaving this world!! And you—*you*, you poor, stupid bastard!—you're gonna keep standing there—*ain't* ya?—holding the bag!!"

"Sir, I—"

"YOU ARE THE DEAD!!!"

And in his drunkenness, and in the desperation of the death of 1932, Theo could not argue with this insane accusation.

"Sure, sir. I'm . . . sure that I am."

"You stupid kid!! What the hell are you gonna do when Sanity has left you?!"

"Well, sir, I—"

"You see that darkness out there?? Moonless, starless

darkness! And the coming dawn, boy—the coming dawn will be *darker still . . ."*

The old man pushed past him, then, to the window on the landing. He kicked the window with his bare feet, blood splattering as the glass crashed around them. Theo tried to hold the old man back, but the man bit at him, so like that strange vagabond Wozzeck in the wilds of Iberia years ago had threatened Guaril, and squirmed out of his grasp. The old man fell the three stories to the ground, crying "WORLD—I **KILL** YOU!!!" before he splashed lifeless on the pavement.

Neighbours woke up in the tenement, and all round the street, babies crying, women shouting, men cursing. The Bullen were called, and the body was scooped up and taken to the city morgue, and from there consigned to a potter's field outside Berlin. No one mourned for the wretch, no relatives, no loved ones, nobody at all even able to identify him in the week that followed. But Theo could never get out of his head the queerness, the insanity of the meeting with a soul he'd heard from almost the very beginning of his adult life, yet had never put a face to—trying to tell him everything in the short span of a minute or two, before whatever unnamed horrors he dealt with came crashing down around him, and pushed him over the edge of that windowpane to his end on their sad little street. It clicked with Theo, in ways he could not name, the convergence of his madness and the madness of the old man, the things Theo had been thinking about over those late-night hours, and the thoughts he'd never know in the old man who had killed himself right in front of him. Theo couldn't do anything for weeks afterwards, as 1932 became 1933. His head was flooded with noises so loud he couldn't sleep, just drifted comatose from dull daydream to dull daydream, the howls of demonic voices, the clanging of tram bells and whistles, the clattering of the machinery in the munitions factory across the street, finally coughing itself back to life, as if anticipating renewed demand for the grenades and mortar-shells it had made long ago. When Theo finally emerged from his coma of uncertainty, the Nazis had won the elections that he and all his anarchist comrades refused to vote in, because no party worthy of their trust ever ran in elections—certainly not now. Hitler was Chancellor of Germany, with the old warmonger veteran, senile old Von Hindenburg, as President.

Theo was sure that the old madman was right in his last utterances. The Nazi swastika, ancient symbol of the sun, had dawned that winter. The long night of Weimar was over now. But the dawn would be darker still . . .

Chapter 23

"But now *is* the time to strike, Katharina! If not now, then *when?!"*

Theo opened his eyes to the bleak light of January 30, 1933, glaring silvery bright and terrible despite the dirty windows and the heavy, soiled crimson curtains. Katya was not in bed with him; nobody was. But even through the suite-double-doors closed but for a crack, Dempsey's booming voice could not be mistaken. Theo heard Katya's voice murmuring low, the way she did when she was thinking aloud. Her voice seemed gradually affirmative.

" . . . Dempsey's right, Oma," Kanalratte's voice came then, "You know it; I know it—we all know it! That fucker's in charge now. How long is that senile old bastard gonna stay president anyway?? He'll up and die in a year or less! And then, Chancellor Hitler'll be President Hitler too!!"

"And then, what d'we got?" Dempsey chimed in. "They're already preparing a camp in Oranienburg—all the Berliners who hate the government are gonna be taken there, held there till the bastards figure out where else to put 'em. I been there before—they got an old brewery they ain't usin' no more, and the fucking SA's takin' it over, and they're gonna make the whole town go and look at it—prisoners on display, like in a *zoo!"*

"It's only a matter of time, now, Katyale," Naomi said to a downcast Katya. "We gotta take action—now, or never."

"Well," Katya said, looking up, "what d'you wanna do? I still got millions' worth of gold in a Swiss bank in Geneva. I could write 'em, tell 'em to send me the lot. We can put it all into . . . incendiaries."

"*Wunderbar, Oma!"* Kanalratte enthused. "Reinhardt's in Cologne, now; he's got connections with the Pirate scene down there—the biggest bunch of us anywhere are there. Quietschend's in Ascona, now, visiting his mum's land. He'll be in touch with your pals, the Tovarisches. There's Pirates all over Germany, now, little handfuls everywhere, in every major town. It'll take us, like, less than a month to arm 'em. Then we could coordinate something— maybe for March 5th, when the new elections Hitler's called for are set, to give him his majority in the Reichstag, and pass that stupid 'Enabling Act' the Nazi fools and all their dumb-ox followers are yellin' about."

"No, no," Dempsey said. "No, it's gotta be before that.

Way before that."

"When, then?" Theo asked. He'd pushed through the crack in the door so softly, none of them had noticed his coming in.

"I dunno, man," Dempsey said. "If I had the stuff to do what I gotta do—I'd say tonight!"

"But we don't have the stuff," Katya said. "It's gonna take me a week to get the money, and another week to get the dynamite, or whatever we need—"

"Leave that to the different groups o' people round the country, Oma," Kanalratte said. "Reinhardt and Quietschend's been working for years on their own 'little projects.' And in each town, there's little groups of boys and gals just like them. If you could send 'em just a little money, Oma, they'll do the rest."

"We gotta strike *before* the government's formed," Dempsey continued to insist. "That's the most important thing."

"Won't they all just blame us more?" Theo asked. "Come down on us harder?"

Dempsey looked rather stupidly ahead of him, and breathed a sigh.

"Theodor, man," he said finally, "what chance do we got o' doin' *anything*, once that Act gets passed? If we don't act now—"

"—If we don't act now," Kanalratte almost shouted, "we'll be just waitin' for 'em to take us all away! I don't wanna grow old, man—I don't see myself past thirty. Fuck! I don't see myself turning twenty!"

"Well, this way, none of us are gonna see much past next month," Theo almost shouted back. Everyone looked at him. They knew him too well to call him a traitor, or a coward. But these were desperate times, and called for desperate actions. They knew it; he knew it. Katya was looking at her lover, too. Her grey eyes reflected his uncertainty, sympathized with it. But when she spoke, she spoke in consensus with her young friends.

"Theo, darling," she said softly. "It might even be a Pyrrhic gesture, a last act of defiance—like suicide, darling—"

"—No, Katharina!" Dempsey said bullheaded. "It's the best thing to do—"

"Please, Dempsey—hear an old woman out! Theo, we've spent the last decade talking, planning, moving here, moving there—playing, and learning, and thinking, and growing—and I wouldn't take any of it back. When we knew Guaril and Johanna, all those years ago—when it was the four of us, together for those seasons—liebling, those were some of my finest moments, my dearest memories. But Guaril's dead; Johanna's dead. *They'll never come back.* The 'twenties are dead. All those things we knew and loved—things these kids never saw—all that's dead, too. We've been licking out wounds too long, Theo. We've been trying to live in the past. Well, I'm going start living right now—for today!—and tomorrow!!"

"It'll be a short day, today," Theo spat, "and there ain't gonna be any tomorrows, Katya, mein schätze."

"Maybe your right, baby. But that fate is ours, *either* way."

"You guys really *are* old, ain't ya?" Kanalratte said, softly, almost disbelievingly. "Life's painful for me now; and it's painful for you guys, too. But at least . . . at least I'm sure of the pain. You guys . . . you guys are like more in pain than even me, because you doubt yourselves so much. You can't even trust yourselves to know pain and call it for what it is. . . . Man, I don't *wanna* get as old as you!"

Theo, who would turn thirty by the instalment of the coming government, just scant weeks from this bleak January, laughed a hollow laugh.

"You ain't gonna, man," he said. "You ain't gonna get any older. I can see that now."

"Well neither the fuck are you! *Face it*, Opa! We've got *nothin'*—nothin' but what kinda noise we're gonna make when we go!"

"See, I don't think it's that bleak," Dempsey said. "I don't think this is the last thing we can do—but the *first* thing! People are angry now—they're mad as hell! It's a powder keg, this Germany—the whole fuckin' Europe! All we are is the spark—"

"—The vanguard," Theo quipped cynically.

"That's *right!* Maybe what you say about communists being, uh, elitist—maybe all that's sense, Theodor. But the communists are organized and ready. You lot ain't organized—that's my biggest problem with you lot."

"Yet," Naomi said, "it's anarchist, to do what the authorities call 'terrorism.' Whether we think of ourselves as a 'vanguard' or not, whether we think the 'masses' are gonna rise up after us, or not—and whether some of us are communist, or anarchist, or just riled up and tired of it all—this thing is still the *only thing to do* . . ."

Theo thought about this. He'd just been dreaming of his father, hearing his father's voice chiding him from beyond the windowpanes that seemed to rattle with his voice upon waking. Theodor's father's voice was shouting about the same kinds of things, as was always with him—even when he still lived, the father said little else. Revolution—right, or wrong? Mass action, mass organizing—right, or wrong? Individual, direct action— 'propaganda of the deed'—was this right, or wrong? Such things filled Theo's waking life, and too haunted his dreams. There were times in debate with flesh-and-blood, real people, that Theodor was really arguing with these voices. He'd begun to see this pattern, and try to break himself of it; but it was still hard. He caught himself now, and tried to reason what he *really* thought about this debate of his friends he just woke up to, and not just react to the voices he'd been dreaming about a moment before.

Slowly, he said, "I don't know what to think any more. I know all the arguments for or against what you guys are planning. I could see our vanguard action inspiring a putsch, then a full-scale rebellion. Yeah, I could see that. But I could just as easily see the repression coming down on us all the harder for it. And, too, I can see a third way: our actions'll do nothing at all in the real world— nothing at all . . . Nothing, maybe, but get us all killed—or stuck in that zoo in Oranienburg, viewed as the bloody museum pieces we already are."

"Speak for yourself, man!" Kanalratte spat. "I ain't *ever* gonna be in anybody's *museum!* No history books'll ever be written about *me!* To *Hell* with history, Theo! We got a chance *right now—* and that's **all we'll ever have!"**

Kanalratte got up then, donned ihre *Mantel* coat and *Mütze* cap, and stormed out. Dempsey sighed again, and prepared to follow sie out.

"Think about it, all right?" he said in parting. "But whatever y'all do, *I'm* gonna do *something.* Some history's gonna be made in the next month—even if it's the *end* o' history."

And with that, Dempsey, too, walked out. Naomi got up.

"Boys, boys, boys," Naomi laughed a little. "I think Dempsey's serious. If he can't get us to help 'im, he'll find somebody else. And I might not seem as much of a hothead as my beau, but I'm at least as riled."

"I am too!" Theo said. "More riled than I can even tell you!"

"Me, too," Katya said softly. "I think being horrendously angry is an occupational hazard of having a working brain in this world."

"Well, I'm gonna go after Dempsey and that other hothead child. Then, I'm going to work, back at that wretched Nachtlokal. . . . I'll be back later, though, okay?"

"You're always welcome, darling."

And Naomi bent down and kissed Katya on each cheek. She went over to Theo, and asked if she could give him a hug.

"Of course," he smiled, and embraced her little body. Then she was gone.

Theo looked to Katya. He found her looking down at her lap again.

"Are you really serious about withdrawing all your money, Katya?"

"What else are we gonna do with it? The way inflation is, and the way we're living now—it'll last just four or five more years anyway. And the way Germany is now, the fucking Nazis'll probably 'nationalize' it all long before then—and you and I will end up in a camp anyway. Our days are numbered, liebling—whatever we do."

Theo collapsed by her feet.

"Yeah, schätze; I know."

"D'you wanna go out with a whimper or a bang, Theo? That's the only decision we've got left. . . . Maybe my parents have the right idea. Get the hell outta here."

"I don't really wanna go to Palestine, Katya."

"Hell! Neither do I! Just because my own country isn't worth living in any more doesn't mean I should go steal somebody else's!"

"Yeah."

"And *everywhere* is somebody else's, Theo. What's that thing that fellow you were reading years ago said, that guy who actually *liked* the rising bureaucratic class?"

"Bruno Rizzi? Yeah, he was saying that it was inevitable they'd take over. Communist, Nazi, Fascist—or even the bigger and bigger governments of the capitalist world. The world's probably going that way, everywhere."

"Yeah. So, what do you do in a world like that? Hide out in the Italian Riviera and look at pretty paintings till the Blackshirts come and drag us away? Or go to America, and wait for the Silvershirts to take over there? There's no place for us now, Theo."

"Yeah; I know."

"I never thought I'd live *this* long. I guess the reason I never committed suicide is that I could never figure out a creative enough way to do it."

Theo smiled. "Creative?"

"Well, yes, suβe. If it *is* in fact your last act—you might as well do something good to make an impression on the audience before the curtain comes down. I mean, there ain't gonna be any curtain calls after *that* performance."

Theo squinted in thought. His father and a dozen other voices were competing to tell him this or that kind of nonsense, as they'd been doing for most of the last six years. He'd be stuck in their narrative till the day he died, he knew now. But the world does not see the stories that go on in your head; they see simply the story *you* fit into in *theirs*. Why not break out of his little narrative of despair by ending that story, and giving himself up to whatever stories later generations might pen him into? Why not *do* something, in thirty years, rather than do *nothing* in fifty-five, or seventy?

And, noted his beloved, to get to fifty-five or seventy in the world that was to come wouldn't be a story worth reading anyway.

"We could really do it, you know," she said looking down at him and up at him at once. "We could both put our heads in that oven, Theo—any time we choose."

"Yeah, but . . . yeah."

"We've been doomed since we started. Wouldn't it be just beautiful if we could *choose* the shape of our own doom, Theo—rather than wait for the ugliness of the world to choose it for us?"

"Yeah. Yeah, it would. Because we both know, love, what it is not to have that choice. Prison and the madhouse. The one way a person really retains the dignity of being a person, is to choose for himself, or herself, when to stop being a person."

"Yeah! Yeah. That's why I really don't care if Dempsey's right, or you are, about the potentials of the People rising up after we do—whatever it is we're gonna do. If they do rise up—beautiful! If they don't, well . . . we'll never know."

"I hope I'm wrong, Katya. I hope Dempsey's right. But, I've spent years trying to convince people to think for themselves, to do for themselves, that they don't need any experts to show them how to do it. And who the hell even read any of those pamphlets, schätzelein? And of those who did, who the hell remembers any of it?"

"You know what, Theo? Maybe that 'individualist' versus 'collectivist' inside joke of that cell I worked with years ago wasn't just nonsense after all. I'm an individualist anarchist, darling, as I know you've always tended to be more toward the collectivist. I say—at the risk of sounding like a traitor—at the risk of losing your respect forever—I say, *Fuck the People,* Theo. Fuck their stupidity and their timidity and their complacency and their apathy and the fact that most of 'em just don't care."

"I could never say that, Katya. But . . . I'd be lying to you if I said the thought's never crossed my mind."

"Freedom is not simply a political thing, Theo. Freedom can mean freedom *from* the political. When I kick a stormtrooper in the nuts, I'm no longer interested in *reaching* him—beyond the reach of my steel-pointed toe in his crotch. With some people— fuck, man, with *most people*—that's as close to 'reaching' them as you're ever gonna get. And, in the final analysis, I'd rather go out making as many of those people's nuts ache as I can. Because, that's all one person can really ever do."

Theo could almost weep at such cynicism. The thing that saved him from despair, over and over and over again in his life— the thing that he argued valiantly with his father and a dozen other ghosts, destined always to argue with them—was the value of Revolution as a spiritual concept. The People were the Good. The People were meant to be Their Own Saviours. But just this once, he let his guard completely down, and listened to Katya. If it were only him and her and a handful of other people in all of Germany— in all the world—and most everybody else was enamoured with hatred and atrocity and the love of the leaders and the safety of their dumb numbers—if he had to throw away the mindset he'd carried through madness and prison and privation and betrayal since he was fifteen years old—then, he could *still* find a way to happiness. He could survive, and maybe even thrive, in a world where he relied on no one but a precious chosen few. No God, No Masters, No Safety in Numbers. No. Nothing now. Nothing but ultimate cynicism, and through that cynicism . . . *freedom.*

And all at once, the voices in his head grew softer, as he realized they, too, were but his fear of being alone. He was not alone. He had just a few comrades; but he could count on them.

Why did he need any more?

"I love you, Katharina."

"I love you, too—my precious, precious fairy-boy, my hot-brother-baby—*my Theodor* . . ."

They made love right there on the floor, fucking wildly and madly, as if they'd never fuck again, as if they meant to die of fucking. When they awoke in the later part of the evening, Katya made a phone call to Sebastien and Nadia in Ascona. She asked them to go to Geneva, and help her arrange for the closing of her account there.

Chapter 24

Arrangements were made over the next weeks, as the speeches of the new Son of God, that Wagnerian vomit Adolf Hitler cried and screamed from the wireless his gospel of hate. There was nothing on the wireless much any more but his voice, crying against the Jews, crying against the Bolshevists (who also, somehow, were Jews), crying just a shade less loudly against the banking elites (who, yes, were nearly always also Jews). It was an old gospel, Hitler's hatreds, old as the Gospel, or almost. The white races of Europe, in order to remain white, had to have a black about to define themselves in opposition to; and the Jews, the Gypsies, the Queers of various stripes, the mad and the physically disabled—and all those who loved them—these were the black smudges on the Nazis' Teutonic blonde purity. Nothing new here, really. Guaril's diagnosis of the madness of Europe rang true a decade after he'd pronounced it: the bane of the European mind was the non-European Other. And so driven toward their white purity were they that the "Aryan races" now had to look within their own populace, their own Continent, to purify themselves still further.

Anti-Semitism was no new song in Europe. The only change in the tune was the air of "science" that had vomited up from the ugly innards of the white-racist beast, to fill its head with a new sophistication. Science, which pronounced things "unfit" where once they'd been unclean. Katya knew the new strain well. She'd spent nearly five years rotting away on a ward of "scientific" isolation from her world for her "mental unfitness." She was in herself nearly every banned category the Nazis hated, wanted to separate from the rest and banish to the nether regions. A Jewess, a Queer, a Madwoman, and, by the Nazis' standards, more than a sympathizer with "Bolshevism" (however untrue that accusation really was). She was doomed twice, thrice over. And so was her Theo, and all the young rebel kids who clung to them now, rallying in the final stand they would take in their lives.

Of course, science could work for them as much as it worked against them. Sebastien and Nadia and their unnamed comrades at their chalet used the monies they withdrew in Katya's name from her bank in Geneva, and got the raw materials that a week of chemical and mechanical and other scientific magic transformed into the cleverest time-bombs anyone had ever known. They were so innocuous, the detonators half-formed, connected with magnets, that they could even be sent through the post with little trouble from customs. And that's what Sebastien did, sending enough magnet-detonators to set off ten bombs of various sizes. The nitroglycerin and dynamite and gunpowder were a little harder to come by, and most of those transactions were done within Germany, as that contraband would most surely be sniffed in a package through the post. Mostly, they had to make due with what they could. From town to town, young, anonymous people, operatives in the unofficial conspiracy, planned to use everything from petrol and kerosene to their own piss in mud to fashion the incendiaries they'd need to do the damage they sought. Here in Berlin, with the Bullen tightening their watch on everything over the month of February, their ranks swelling with former stormtroopers and other Nazi thugs, with all the zealotry of a newly-vindicated nascent ruling class, Dempsey and the others put their heads together to see what they might use. The munitions factory across the street from the slum salon, like others round town, was guarded all hours of the day and night, as were most construction sites round town where dynamite and other incendiaries might have been gotten. They all decided not to use the detonators or the few vials of nitroglycerin they'd bartered for on the black market, deciding to save all that for some future action. Somebody Dempsey was in contact with hit on a wonderful solution to the problem: celluloid, in the film capitol of Europe, was easy to come by, and hiring themselves out to clean up the chopping floors of editing rooms all over Berlin, Dempsey's shadowy circle of communists whom the Pirates never met, gathered a pile of it all together by the third week of February, storing it at Katya's and Theo's flat.

Theo laughed looking at the closetful of old films, including a few reels of what appeared the passé genre he'd seen mocked and mangled more than ten years ago in the very room he stood in now.

"Another fucking Otto Gebuhr flick," he chuckled, looking through the frames to see the now old man's face. "Surprised that fuck's still breathin'. You know, Katya, my love? I do believe this last shit's straight from my sister's studio! Yeah, she'd be just the kind of person who'd help make films about German heroes from the caveman days. Otto fucking Gebuhr! Fire's too good for this shit . . ."

Theo was won over now, agreeing with Katya and all that the time had come for action, however misguided and ineffective he still thought it would be. And things were encouraging, he had to admit. Hamburg, Leipzig, Munich, Frankfurt, Essen, Dusseldorf, Oberhaussen, Cologne—all of these towns had little pockets of Pirates and their allies, just waiting for a signal from "auntie." Their "rich auntie," who'd sent off the Berlin Pirates with loads of what incendiaries they'd managed to steal or buy or brew from scratch all round Berlin, to bike with their backpacks full on a week-long cross-country tour through the wilds and fens of Deutschland. Other towns were rumoured also to be in league. But really, all Katya and Theo and Dempsey and Naomi could count on was Berlin—for it was they who *were* Berlin at that moment. Auntie made her calls, when her "niece" or "nephew" found *ihren Weg,* ihren way round to Cologne and connected with Reinhardt and his pals down there, and both kids patched a wire to the slum salon saying the single word "DON'T." This was a play on words, for in the lingo of telegrams, everything is ended with "STOP." Thus, the message was *DON'T STOP.*

This was their cue.

"Okay," Dempsey breathed in the darkening afternoon of February 27th, 1933. "My pals'll be here in an hour, guys. They're gonna bring the truck round. Then we can bring these crates of film down there."

"You got the fire-lighters, kiddo?" Naomi asked.

"Yeah, I got 'em. I got 'em all."

"I really wish we coulda met these 'friends' o' yers, Dempsey, man," Theo said. "It's weird, relying on people outside our circle to do what the circle has been planning, just among us."

"Yeah, Theodor, but it couldn't be helped. As it is, they ain't even gonna see the inside o' this place. That's to protect you lot. And these pals o' mine—communist comrades I met a couple months back—they're good people, man. But they ain't ones to trust any easier than you lot."

"My pretty, tough little boy," Naomi smiled on her boyfriend, "the go-between. The one who takes *all* the risks . . ."

Dempsey just smiled at this.

"Somebody's gotta, kid," he said finally. "And it might as well be me."

Naomi embraced him then, and a small tear was in her eye. She knew somehow that, whether the fire was successful or not, whether Dempsey got away or not, somehow she knew: she'd never see her beau again.

"Don't cry, kid," the young, boxer's face smiled to his pretty girlfriend, who was trying to smile through her tears. "No, no. We gotta be tough, now. Otherwise . . . otherwise, I'm afraid I'll lose my nerve."

Naomi smiled and sniffed back her sobs. She wiped her eyes, and offered her teary hand for him to kiss.

"Salt's good for ya, kiddo," she giggled, some private joke of theirs. Dempsey chuckled gratefully, and licked the tears off her hand. Then he kissed her lips like a young boy with his first love. Perhaps Naomi really *was* that for him . . . but nobody would ever know; Naomi would never tell.

Hugging her little body with his big, clumsy arms, Dempsey turned then and picked up four big crates of celluloid, stacked higher than his head, and made his way down the hallway outside to the backstairs. Theo and Naomi and Katya followed with two or three crates each, making it down into a back alley just as a dark-windowed, beat up Willy's Overland pulled up to where they were standing. Dempsey put his big, thick body between the car and his friends, as if to protect their identities from people Theo began to sense not even he really trusted. A sick feeling began to well up in Theodor then, as if his young friend were heading straight into a trap. But it was too late now.

Dempsey, with an almost herculean strength, slugged all the crates into the back of the Willy's Overland, looking back at them as if to say, *"You lot—**don't come too close, now . . .**"*

When he was done, Dempsey smiled a brave smile to them and waved his hand once. Then he jumped into the back seat, and the car spun away before he'd even fully closed the door.

Now, it was just a question of waiting. A long, long wait that night . . .

The scheduled time for the great event was half past nine in the evening. Whatever transpired elsewhere, the Berlin target went down without a hitch. Dempsey was supposed to leave town for a week that night, and return to a rendezvous point he'd worked out with Naomi. She did not tell where that place was, and nobody pressed her. But the morning edition of the papers on the last day of February had headlines of what happened, and reading it, Naomi wept to know that her secret meeting point with her boy was as irrelevant as some crater on the moon—Dempsey would as likely be there in a week as where he'd worked out with Naomi. The shady pals Dempsey had chosen to work with were not mentioned in the paper; only one "Marinus van der Lubbe" had been apprehended, just a block away from the Reichstag, without his shirt on in the cold. He'd confessed to starting the fire there, though even the papers said there were too many inflammables, twenty bundles of which hadn't even gone off, for any person to have acted alone. It was the first time anybody besides Naomi had ever heard Dempsey's real name.

Nothing showed up about any other place that was supposed to go up, not in Cologne, not in Hamburg, not in Leipzig or Dusseldorf or any other places. Doubtless some of the smaller towns had seen some action, but in the glare of the fire in the most important building in the most important city in Germany, no lesser light could shine. Within hours of the fire, arrests were being made. It was as if somebody was in the know somewhere in the halls of government, and had already prepared the mass arrests beforehand. Again, the shadiness of those "pals" of Dempsey turned Theo's stomach. No word came from anywhere. Could all the kids have been arrested last night?

Katya and Theo and Naomi wasted no time. Before noon, they were already far outside Berlin, heading down to Bavaria, to a little cottage Katharina had stayed in a few stolen nights over a summer of her youth, down a lonely country road from one of her family's summer estates. That estate had been burned to the ground by an angry, fascist mob along with a lot of other things connected to her family and a dozen other Jewish bourgeois families in the area. Katya knew, a little guiltily, but also with a certain perverse pleasure, that the publicity round her trial three years ago had had something to do with the riot at her ancestral summer home. She wouldn't have gone there by choice anyway, not even to escape the repression. But the little cottage she'd found wandering away from her ugly family when she was just twelve years old, once belonging to some peasant woman who was said to be a witch who back in the nineteenth century committed suicide (or was spirited away by the Devil, or the fairies, or the gypsies, as other folk said), and who still was said to haunt the place—this place where she'd escaped with her family's stable-boy over a few dark and stormy nights, and passed her first milestone on the long, winding road of her erotic life in his arms—this place, she'd go again. She'd made sure to let the people whom she cared about most in the world know the location of the place. The Pirates, mobile all over the Continent on their sleek-framed bicycles, would all gather there soon—if any of them were still at liberty.

Theo, Katya, and Naomi made their way down there by auto, a nondescript old flivver Naomi had purchased just two days before with money Katya had given her, under a false name. They made their way down by the end of the day, passing the burnt-out ruin of the old Von Rosen estate, then down obscure side roads through farm and forest and feral land to the little cottage in the woods, which seemed as much a ruin.

"Here, kids," smiled Katharina as she jumped out of the driver's seat onto the glorious, sweet-smelling mud, softened by an early spring rain. "Here's where we die . . ."

And Theo walked through the country as if he were already in the afterlife. Naomi thought of her body buried beneath this mud, or cremated and scattered here—maybe in that creek, flowing down the way—maybe over in that ravine further on . . . Dempsey, her best friend, was lost now. They'd kill him for sure.

The three prepared a vigil in the wilds, giving their friends a week, no more, to show, before they would make their final move.

They only vaguely knew what that move would be . . .

Chapter 25

A week passed, and there was no groundswell of revolution in Germany. Maybe times had changed. Maybe revolutions weren't to happen in this land any more. But the wireless they'd brought kept them abreast of what was going on. Right or wrong, Dempsey had shaken the rotten government up, but good. History had definitely been made; and the wheels of history were just a little jolted by Dempsey's brave little spanner.

The paranoia of the government, knowing they did not rule absolutely, that there were untold thousands—maybe millions—who were not goose-stepping along with their new order, and were prepared to take action against them—got quickly translated into fear of Communist Revolution. If the KPD had been true revolutionaries, and not the bankrupt traitors to revolution the bureaucrats of the Third International had so obviously become, they'd have made the fight the few comrades of the slum salon and the Pirates round the country had fired the first shot in. But, no, no. Alas, the people did not rise. Alas, the blame was put on the Communist Party, and not the ordinary people, the truer rebels, that had really done the deed. And, Theo's worst fears were borne out: instead of the spark of conflagration, the fire in the Reichstag signalled the beginning of the police-state in truth. The KPD comrades did little to defend themselves against the mass of arrests which swept through Germany that week. Mostly, they went like sheep to the slaughter. And slaughtered most all of them were.

A bicyclist came banging down the dirt road leading to the haunted cabin in the latest twilight, on the day the elections the monster Hitler had called were held, March 5th. The elections went as everybody expected they would: a plurality for the Nazis, with the slack taken up by the German National People's Party, the Catholic Centre Party, and the scattered remnants of various middle class parties—all of which supported the general push toward the authoritarian regime. The Communists were banned from the election, and the Socialists, the only opposition left, were all harassed by Brownshirts that morning before they could take their seats. No opposition made any meaningful stand in that week. Hitler carried the day; the Enabling Act passed with an easy majority in the parliament that had to meet at the old Opera House, the Reichstag still a ruin. The bicyclist was fully aware of all the parliamentary falderal, and cared not a jot for it. Kanalratte skidded to a stop, then stood with ihr *Fahrrad* bicycle in the dust, and waited.

Theo came out right away, with Katya and Naomi behind him. They embraced the rebel child in the moonlight, even before sie had dismounted the bike, laughing joyfully to see a comrade yet alive. Kanalratte threw ihr bicycle down in the dirt, and turned to them. Sie had been through a lot over that week; it was evident in the expression on ihr face. Sie looked to them, and shivered.

"Come, tell us," invited Katya. "Tell us all the bullshit in the world. . . . You're home now."

"Yeah," Kanalratte said. "I suppose this place, in the middle of nowhere, is as much a home as I'm ever likely to get. . . . They've taken Erich."

"Erich Mühsam?" Theo asked.

"Yeah. They got him in the first hours after the fire. Fucking bastards. It's almost like they knew in advance of it. Fucking, fucking bastards . . ."

And Theo thought too much of Kanalratte, too much of Erich, too much of all the others, to say what he'd been thinking for the last week: that Dempsey had been set up, that his "comrades" were nothing but government agents all along. No, Theo couldn't say that. Yet, everyone else seemed to know it, then, too.

Katya hugged Kanalratte again, thinking to the elderly arms Erich had embraced her with, just a year and a half ago, in a season much like this one, cold, wet, between death and life. She knew sie was not used to the affection, but she offered it anyway, knowing both of them, sie and her, needed a hug badly then, even if neither felt like admitting it. She let go, and waited for the tough, pretty person to make *ihr Testament*, what sie had seen and done in the week since the greatest event in the radical world in a generation had gone down, for better or worse. Kanalratte had much more to say.

"Reinhardt's been taken," sie said. "All the Cologne Pirates've been taken. Quietschend's been deported—dunno even where he is. Could be in Switzerland—could be in bloody Japan. All over this bumsen Deutschland—Essen, Leipzig, Dusseldorf, Oberhaussen, Frankfurt, Hamburg—all over, man, they've taken us, or disappeared us. There must've been a hundred arrests of our people. God knows what'll happen now—and God's a senile old bastard, like useless old Von Hindenburg—destined for rot. I just got out o' there by the skin of my teeth . . ."

Kanalratte said it was over. And the comrades round sie did not argue with the appraisal. They knew then, that whatever they might have done, or not done, it all would have ended up the same. At least they'd tried. The world was doomed now; they all knew it. And they, the forward-thinking, along with the countless ignorant bastards of Deutschland, were doomed right along with it. The Nazi dawn would last a thousand years . . .

"They took Erich," Kanalratte said again, bitterly, as if sie had reasons of ihre own to mourn the old man as more than just a comrade and friend. "He's being held in some cold, dark cell in Oranienburg. The whole of Germany—all the people that matter—will soon be there, right there with 'im. . . . What are we gonna do, man?"

Katya looked to Theo, to Naomi.

"Well," she said, "I've still got enough for a second class ticket for us all. . . . Why not get it, now? Why not divert the flood, if only for a week or two? What d'you say, everybody?"

They knew it was the end. That old bastard, that Britisher poet of the Lost Generation, celebrated by every clever bourgeois and petty-bourgeois over the whole of Europe, the clever wisdom of the powerless, that this generation would go out with a whimper and not a bang, the apocalyptic forecast in a world that that anti-Semite poet could only himself partially appreciate, so bound down by his own ugly prejudices—T.S. Eliot was too busy at his banking day-job to ever understand the folk who would defy his cynical prediction. The four of them standing there in the after-twilight, feral forest of Bavaria, decided to throw a last wrench into the gears and wheels of history—even if the result was but a postponement of the inevitable. If Oranienburg was where they were taking everybody, all the rebel people of Berlin—just like Dempsey, that poor ill-fated fool, that hero and saint to them all, said they would—then they'd toss their spanner there. With uncharacteristic determination and certainty, the anarchists hampered by age came together with those hampered only by inexperience, and decided together their collective fate.

They would stop the trains.

The last of Katya's money, the last vestige of her bourgeois privilege in the world, was burned that night, all the billions of useless Papiermarks mingling with infinitely more valuable, but in the end just as useless Rentenmarks and Reichsmarks—gold and silver, rusting, burning—to keep them warm in the spooky cottage in the night. The fire breathed and glowed and spread over the course of the night, till by morning the whole house was on fire. The four left the place before dawn had fully cleared the trees, leaving the blaze to smoulder for hours and hours after they'd left, the second to last conflagration they'd leave as their calling card in the world. By the time they'd gotten their tickets for a train going north, the whole world seemed ablaze . . .

The journey to Oranienburg would take just an hour or two. They piled on as the most nondescript of commuters in the little flag-stop in the small Bavarian town near Katya's family's old estate, their plans hidden on their falsely cheerful faces. They found an unoccupied second class compartment, just the four of them, a proud, militant-nephalist androgyne, a widower of an ill-fated romance with the most sincere activist in a generation, and two veterans of wars too deep and awful to have a name. These last two, looking to one another, spoke softly of beauty and truth, and a whole host of sweet nonsense, holding their magnetized detonators in a special place. Kanalratte and Naomi would take the watches of the front and the back of the train, a train loaded with SA stormtroopers and other ugly, horrid bastards of the new order. This passage of the train was to put in place the staff of the first concentration camp of the new Germany, the first apparition of the inexorable Nazi dawn. The prisoners had come before, and would come by the droves after. But *this* train . . . this train was the luxury passage of the oppressors, picking up bright-faced young SA-men from all the brightly fascist towns of southern and central Germany as the train thundered north. The four comrades had heard of it from the wireless, a minor point in a minor newscaster's minor news of the day: *The staff of our Führer's new detention centre for the People's enemies will be arriving in Oranienburg in the next hours; citizens are encouraged to welcome them at the Oranienburg train station, and view the dirty Bolshevist radicals who shall be displayed there . . .*

Naomi left the second class compartment before Kanalratte, hugging and kissing Katya and Theo before she went.

"I love you guys," she said, and each of them loved her. So much could have been said; so much had yet to be said between them. But it was done, now. It was all over.

Naomi headed with single purpose to the head of the train,

to the engine. Her plans were dubious to the couple who loved one another like no other, who loved her too as no other. Something about the luger pistol she carried in her gaudy handbag, one that had belonged to her uncle, stolen from a czarist officer. Enough bullets in it for the company of engineers and firemen, and one left over.

Kanalratte did not want hugs and kisses. And the old Opa and Oma respected this. Theo could not help himself from offering his hand, though, for the littlest touch of tenderness, which the tough androgyne returned.

"Funny," Kanalratte sneered, "how a gesture of mutual distrust can be the closest two people can hope to be."

"Yeah," Theo said, clinging a second longer than custom called for, "funny how that is."

"I'll do my part, Opa," Kanalratte said. "—*Theo*. Thanks, old brother, for everything."

"Thank *you*," Theo said. Then the sewer rat disappeared down the little tunnel of the second class corridor, heading for the guard's van, and the host of documents that were being brought to Oranienburg, to prepare for the flood of prisoners soon to follow. Kicking an old stormtrooper in the nuts, then ending him with a shove of his nose deep into his skull with the heel of *ihre Armee-Boot*, a boot some duped soldier died wearing in the trenches at Passchendaele, then had ripped off him by someone whose own boots had been stolen—boots stolen and stolen and stolen again—stolen last by sie—the sewer rat broke past the SA corpse and into the guard's van, and then danced on the files and records of the prisoners at the camp now and the prisoners to come. Sie made a ticker-tape parade of the papers and photos, watching it all disappear into the gloom of the afternoon behind the swiftly moving train.

"Go," sie laughed, as the last of the documents flew away, "go on—fertilize the flowers . . . same as the rest of us . . ." And Kanalratte followed the stream of confetti, no one ever knowing if sie landed safely in the dust beside the tracks.

Theo turned to Katya. Their cabin was two opposing, cushioned benches. They laughed lightly about which they'd choose for their final act, and decided on nothing particular. They fell together on one or another, going forward or going backward, it mattered little. They wore their heavy greatcoats loaded with dynamite and gunpowder and nitroglycerin, knowing that whatever lay ahead in the next moments, there'd be enough to do the thing they'd come there to do. They kissed, passionately, and worked the magic of the magnets into the magic of one another.

Katya had considered her final act, that act that would bring down the curtain, that would leave no prospect of a curtain call. And her Theo loved her, and would give his all to the summation. They kissed, as they had when they first met, more than ten years before, when a demonstration destroyed led to the beginning of their friendship, that kiss in that back alley, that feigned tryst that deterred the Bullen and all the authorities when they were young and nigh virginal in what they knew of the world. They lived that kiss again, in the twilit cabin, knowing that what they were about to do would make a dent in the iron scheme of history, yet would never live in that grim testament beyond the breathy heat of their bodies entwining now. Theory, history—none of it mattered now. Now, all was the entrancing scents and tastes and touch of their bodies entwining, the explosive power of their union enough to propel them into the forefront of a history they'd never read. All was useless now, all pointless and foolish in the grim eye of the Great Man, the Bismark, the Lenin, the Hitler—all the figureheads, the touchstones later generations would call up from the depths of pre-memory to sanction what they felt to be true, but could never prove. Who knew what the 'twenties meant, what the 'thirties, what Germany or Weimar or the whole wide, queer world? Everything faded now into primal thrusts, delicious dancing of lover and loved. And the magnets clicked and made love as their flesh made love, gathering friction and heat, as the train sped closer and closer to the Oranienburg station.

"Theo, darling," Katharina breathed as she came close to orgasm in his arms, *"d'you think anyone'll ever care?"*

"No," her lover breathed. *"No, Katya, love. Nobody'll know. We'll be forgotten—nobody we love'll survive this."*

She closed her beautiful blue-grey eyes, and laughed in triumph.

"Then—I don't care! . . . Fuck me, Theodor; fuck me like you're the last of your kind on this earth—the last of the fucking kind! The last single, solitary person who lives and breathes still!!"

"I love you, Katharina!" he gasped—**"All my life—I've loved you! As long as I've been truly me—it's been for the love of you! That's why I've even stayed here this long—through all this mad Scheiße!"**

"I've loved you the same, Theodor! We're the same—you

and me!! Do you feel us?"

"Yes!!"

"Do you feel it?! It'll be over in ten seconds, Theo—but for us—for us!—it's FOREVER!!"

And he breathed her in, and she breathed him in—deep, drunken breaths—all the cells of their bodies coming together—all fucking at once. As they pushed deeper into one another, tongue in tongue, lips in lips, sex in sex—the wires of their explosive, magnetized realities pushed together, too—their delicious friction warming them and warming them and the explosives to which they were wired—until they were hot enough to spark.

They roared and laughed into a final silence. Magnets fused, sparks flew, and a train of a hundred Nazi Browshirts never arrived at their destination at Oranienburg, the first of hundreds of camps for the annihilation of those unfit for this world. The monsters that ran this madness, this forward-goosestep-march of history, civilisation, and sense, were sidetracked for one moon's journey round the globe by the direct action of desperate people. Doomed from the start, the boy and the girl, children of a lost generation, lived their doom defiant and happy.

Of course, life went on beyond that explosion. Like an insect, worming its way through the trash in the darkness, human life survived, survives. Erich Mühsam was the last of the old comrades, he and Dempsey. Both were already there at Oranienburg, and both took hope from the explosion down the tracks, but a mile and a verst from the town. Dempsey was executed in the courtyard of a Leipzig prison where he was transferred after languishing in Oranienburg for months, beaten, tortured, but never naming any who helped him burn the hated Reichstag. He was beheaded for High Treason, a charge that would hang on his name for decades to come, till a court of another Germany, a Germany that had forgotten the thousand years of the new Reich and the millions who faded over the millennia of its dozen years, overturned the verdict, and exonerated Dempsey in the eighth year of a later century. What crime was it, the great grandchildren's generation would say, to strike at the heart of a corrupt and criminal regime?

Erich hung on for a month after Dempsey. Beaten, starved, they made him dig his own grave in a mummery of execution. They kicked him till he lost most all his teeth, then they took a picture of him for their papers, so he, bearded, wild-haired, with a swastika branded on his forehead by the bastards, would look every part the "Jewish, Bolshevist Menace." On the night he died, the stormtroopers gathered round and forced him on his knees before their ugly flag of the dead sun. They commanded him to sing the *Horst-Wessel-Lied,* their fighting song named for a martyred pimp and murdering stormtrooper, killed by a communist—the new anthem of the land. Toothless, spitting blood, old Erich turned his eyes to the moon, and phrased a song of defiance instead:

> *Arise, ye victims of starvation—arise ye wretched of the Earth! For justice thunders Condemnation—A BETTER WORLD'S IN BIRTH!*

And they kicked him till he was unconscious. As he breathed his last, they hanged him from the stall of a latrine, and told the world he'd killed himself in the night. The cowards wouldn't even own up to his murder. But everyone—all round the world—*everyone knew.*